Slim Forever

The French Way

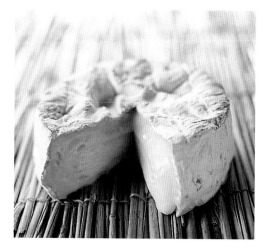

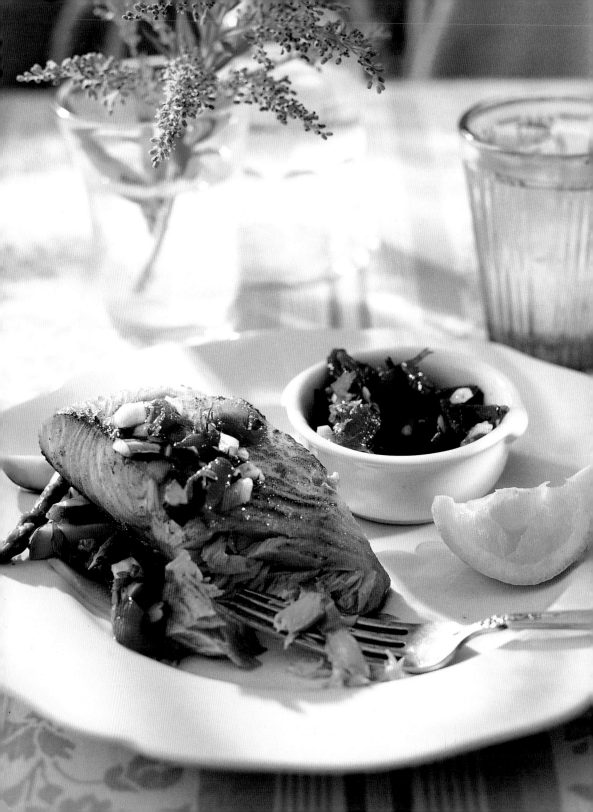

Slim Forever
The French Way

Michel Montignac

For more information visit the
Montignac Universal Official Website
at www.montignac.com or the
Montignac Boutique & Café website
at www.montignacshop.co.uk

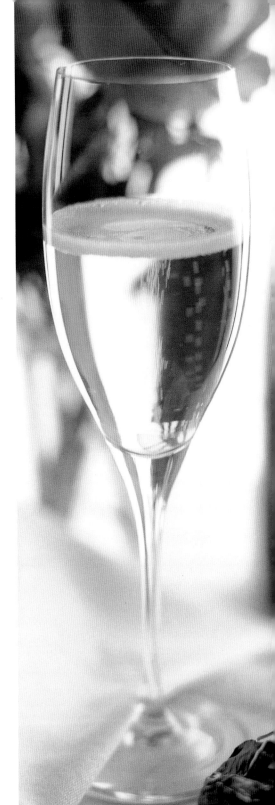

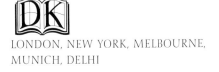

LONDON, NEW YORK, MELBOURNE,
MUNICH, DELHI

Project Editor Shannon Beatty
Project Designer Jo Grey
Senior Editor Jennifer Jones
Project Art Editor Sara Robin
Managing Editors Stephanie Farrow, Penny Warren
Managing Art Editor Marianne Markham
Publishing Manager Gillian Roberts
Art Director Carole Ash
Publishing Director Mary-Clare Jerram
DTP Designer Sonia Charbonnier
Production Controller Elizabeth Warman
Photographer Kate Whitaker
U.S. Editor Nichole Morford
US.. Recipe Adapter Peggy Fallon

First American edition 2006

Published in the United States by
DK Publishing
375 Hudson Street
New York, NY 10014

06 07 08 09 10 10 9 8 7 6 5 4 3 2 1

Published in Great Britain by Dorling Kindersley, Limited.

A catalog record for this book is available from the Library of Congress.

ISBN-13: 978-0-7566-2120-9
ISBN-10: 0-7566-2120-8

Color reproduction by GRB, Italy
Printed and bound by South China Printing Co. Ltd, China

Discover more at

www.dk.com

Contents

Foreword

Twenty years ago, when I published my first book on weight watching, losing weight was basically an aesthetic concern. In 1997, however, after the World Health Organization raised the alarm and decreed that obesity was a health risk and that it had become an epidemic affecting people worldwide, weight control became a public health consideration.

Meanwhile, long before the end of the second millennium, nutritionists and other diet authorities had started to address this problem. For 50 years, they had been trying to make us feel guilty by telling us that, if we were overweight, it was simply because we ate too much—particularly too much fat—and did not exercise enough. However, more recently published epidemiological studies indicate exactly the opposite. These studies show that, since 1960, people in the West have been reducing their daily calorific intake (particularly fats) by 25 to 35 percent and that, paradoxically, obesity has risen by 400 percent during the same period.

Hundreds of scientific studies carried out during the past 25 years show that our hormones, and not calories, are at the heart of obesity. The true cause is hyperinsulinism—a chronic and excessive secretion of insulin, a key metabolic hormone—a condition which is the last stage of a metabolic chain reaction triggered by certain foods—principally high glycemic carbohydrates.

Throughout the past several decades "the dietary landscape" in Western societies has changed considerably. To begin with, highly processed foods, practically unknown to our ancestors, have been progressively introduced into our food chain, to the

Right, opposite: on this diet you can eat cheese and drink wine and still lose weight.

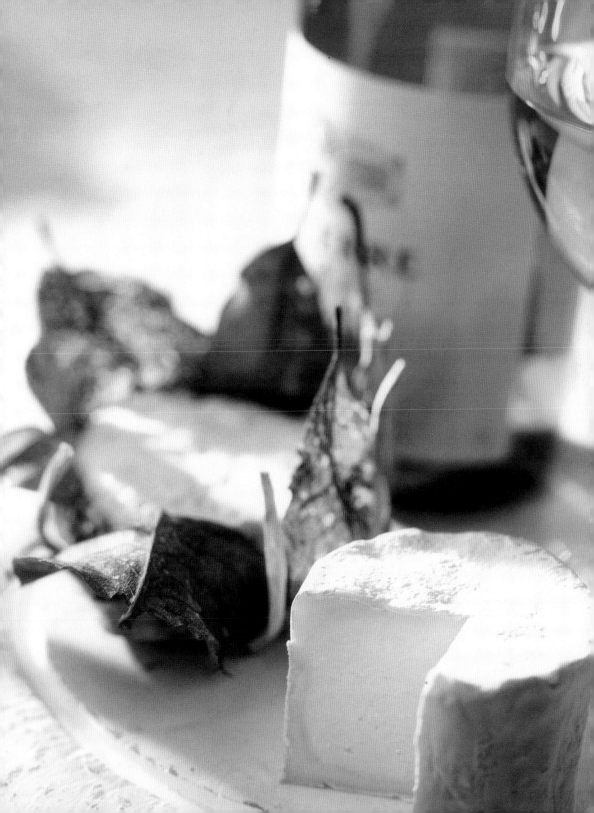

point of becoming an essential part of our daily lives. Furthermore, the transformation of our everyday food through industrial processing and production has significantly modified the quality of the food we eat.

The nature of the food we eat nowadays stimulates metabolic reactions that channel this food into fatty reserves and jeopardize our bodies' normal energy-burning processes. This is why, on the basis of numerous scientific studies, I have designed a dietary model aimed at teaching people to choose those foods that trigger metabolic responses that allow our bodies to burn food as energy instead of storing it as fat.

Although this applies to all food categories, our choice of carbohydrates is especially decisive. Unfortunately, misconceptions regarding carbohydrates remain rife, despite evidence over the past 25 years that the notion of slowly digested carbohydrates and rapidly digested carbohydrates is erroneous, since there is no physiological basis for this belief. As far as our metabolism is concerned, there is no real distinction between "simple" and "complex" carbohydrates. Scientifically, the only criterion that serves to distinguish one carbohydrate from another is its glycemic index (GI). This concept is largely unknown, even though it was proven to be true over 25 years ago.

I had the opportunity to hit upon this concept while the eminent diabetes scientists who discovered it were struggling to have it accepted in their domain, where it is still only marginally taken into consideration. I decided to apply the idea to weight loss. The results of my experiments were so extraordinary that it became the key element in my recommendations on nutrition. I thus had the honor of becoming the first author in the world to propose the concept

"the only criterion that serves to distinguish one carbohydrate from another is its glycemic index (GI)."

of the glycemic index in relation to weight loss. Many other diet books have followed on my heels. But as they have a lack of background in the GI area, they often broadcast distorted, and even incorrect, information.

For decades overweight people have listened to official dieticians, who recommend counting calories and following a low-fat diet, a recipe which has failed over and over again. Inspired by the Atkins diet, several opinion leaders have in recent years declared carbs the real evil. They have switched from one extreme to the other, recommending very low-carb diets. However, people quickly become bored eating this way and may develop cardiovascular problems in the long term. This is why my eating plan is the only perfectly balanced diet. It suggests the right carbs and the right fats.

The goal of this book is to give people who want to lose weight unbiased information regarding an original nutritional concept that has not only proven to be extremely effective, but has also time and again been confirmed by subsequent scientific studies.

I wish you an enlightening discovery.

Michel Montignac

"my eating plan is the only perfectly balanced diet. It suggests the right carbs and the right fats."

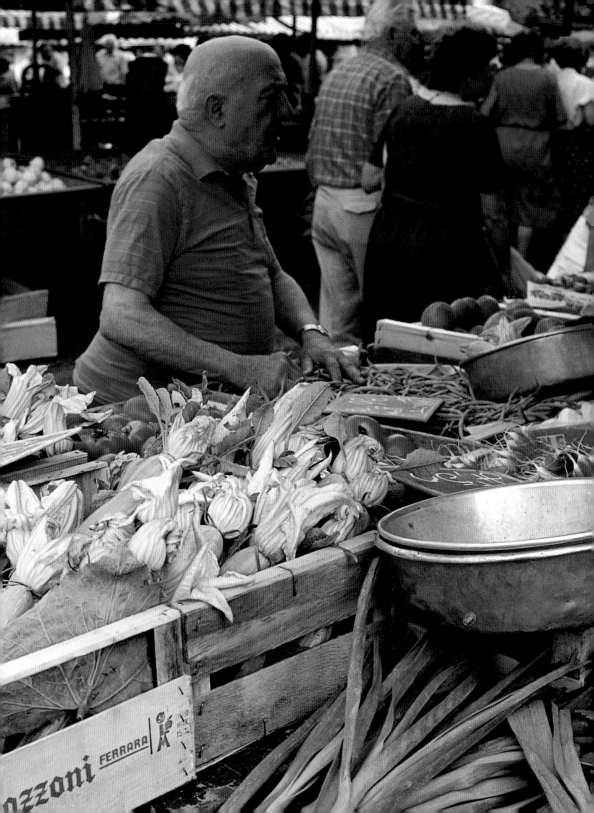

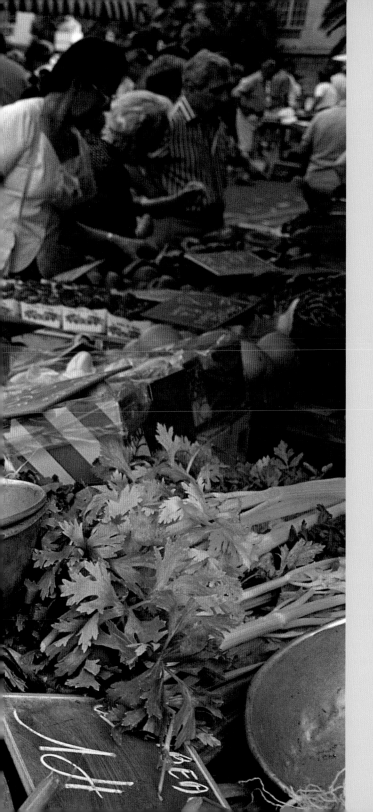

WHY IT WORKS

The calorie myth

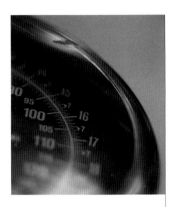

The low-calorie approach to losing weight is based on a simple model that ignores the complexity of the human metabolism. At best it is simplistic; at worst it is dangerous because it can permanently undermine your health. Look around and you will see that the plump, the portly, even the obese, are precisely those who count their calories with the greatest fervor.

THE YO-YO EFFECT

The so-called yo-yo effect describes the invariable outcome of low-calorie diets. It refers to the uncontrollable up and down of a dieter's weight after he or she returns to a normal calorific intake. This occurs because low-calorie diets can reduce the basal metabolic rate (the rate at which the body uses calories when at rest) by up to 50 percent, which translates into significant weight gain when normal eating habits are resumed.

THE BOILER METAPHOR

Nutritionists tend to portray the body as a boiler using up energy in the form of calories. If the calories eaten exceed the calories used by the body, then we gain weight. The calories not "burned" by the body are stored as body fat. The problem with this model is that it ignores the way the body uses calories. Contrary to what many people believe, obese people do not eat more calories than slim people. Medical studies have shown the difference in calorific intake between slim, average, and overweight people is, most of the time, insignificant.

The survival instinct

Anyone who has ever followed a low-calorie diet knows that there is an initial period of quick weight loss. This is because the body is accustomed to receiving a certain number of calories and when this number decreases, the body will use an alternative source, such as body fat, to make up the difference. Early weight loss is followed by a plateau, and most of us find it impossible to maintain our weight in the long term.

In response to receiving less food, the body responds as though it has been threatened with starvation, and gradually reduces its energy output so that it will not have to use fat reserves for energy in the future. The result is that the body's basal metabolic rate (the rate at which the body uses energy when at rest) decreases by as much as 50 percent and no further weight loss occurs. In other words, low-calorie diets actually slow down your metabolism (*see chart, below*). This reduced basal metabolic rate leaves your body vulnerable to rapid and excessive weight gain once you come off the low-calorie diet.

Formula for obesity

In the Western world, the low-calorie approach to weight loss has become a part of our culture, institutionalized at every level despite the fact that a reduction in calories can drastically lower metabolic activity. This means that after following a low-calorie diet, any return to normal calorific intake will bring about weight gain.

The sad paradox is that the more you try to reduce your calorie intake, the faster you will put on weight after you come off your diet. In addition, people who embark on low-calorie diets often suffer from fatigue and an impaired immune system, leaving them susceptible to infection and illness. My diet plan, which does not require you to weigh or measure quantities, offers you a better, less restrictive way to lose weight permanently.

" the plump, the portly, even the obese, are precisely those who count their calories with the greatest fervor."

The cross of the undernourished

This graph shows the history of a woman starting with an average daily calorific intake of 2800. Before going on her first diet, her weight is a stable 220 pounds. As you can see, each time she goes on a low-calorie diet, she goes through a cycle of losing, stabilizing, and regaining her weight. Each successive diet is accompanied by a small weight gain beyond her initial weight. After a few low-calorie diets, she subsists on less than 1000 calories a day and weighs more than 243 pounds.

weight in pounds	NORMAL DIET	1ST DIET	2ND DIET	3RD DIET	4TH DIET
243lb					
198lb					
	2800 cal	2000 cal	1500 cal	1000 cal	800cal

Where does the weight come from?

People gain weight not because they eat too much, but because they eat the wrong foods, which in turn wreak havoc on the body in the form of obesity, diabetes, and cardiovascular disease. Undoubtedly, the strong culinary traditions of the French have made it easier for them to resist the spread of the fast-food culture and lifestyle.

THE CARBOHYDRATE CONNECTION

In the war on weight, the only food group that really concerns us is carbohydrates, and they are the main subject of this book. Carbohydrates are made up of units of sugar (*for more on carbohydrates, see pp32–37*). Insulin, a hormone secreted by the pancreas, plays a vital role in the metabolism of carbohydrates.

During digestion, the sugars in carbohydrates are broken down into simple sugars, mainly glucose, which is then absorbed into the bloodstream. Glycemia is the scientific term for the amount of glucose in the blood, or blood sugar level.

The presence of glucose in the bloodstream triggers the pancreas to release insulin, which enables glucose to pass from the blood into the cells of the body. Once it is in the cells, glucose is burned together with oxygen to create energy.

In a healthy person's body, any excess glucose is converted into glycogen (a complex carbohydrate), which is held in the muscles and liver as a short-term energy reserve. During the course of the day, and specifically between meals when our energy reserves start to drop, the pancreas triggers the hormone glucagon to turn glycogen back into glucose. This process ensures that the body maintains a steady blood-sugar level throughout the day.

"the strong culinary traditions of the French have made it easier for them to resist the spread of the fast-food culture and lifestyle."

The hyperglycemic-hypoglycemic cycle

When you eat high-sugar carbohydrates, it destabilizes your blood-sugar levels and traps your body into a vicious cycle of hyperglycemia and hypoglycemia. This happens because eating a high-sugar carbohydrate causes the level of sugar, or glucose, in your blood to rise far above normal. This is called hyperglycemia. In response, your pancreas floods the bloodstream with insulin. This usually excessive amount of insulin chases the glucose out of the bloodstream, which causes blood-sugar levels to fall far below normal. This state, known as hypoglycemia, makes you feel hungry and shaky, which prompts you to reach for a high-sugar snack, and the cycle begins again.

Eat high-sugar food, which triggers a spike in blood-sugar level (hyperglycemia)

High blood-sugar level stimulates the pancreas to secrete a large amount of insulin

Excess insulin chases too much sugar, or glucose, out of the bloodstream

Lack of glucose causes significant drop in blood-sugar level (hypoglycemia)

Body feels shaky, so you reach for a high-sugar snack

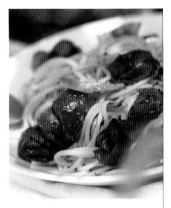

PASTA

Spaghetti, depending on what it is made from and how it is cooked, can be either a high-sugar carbohydrate or a low-sugar one. If you always choose pasta in its least glycemic form (*see pp64–65*), it will not lead to high blood-sugar levels, or hyperglycemia.

So where does it all go wrong?

As we have seen, eating carbohydrates causes the level of sugar in the bloodstream to rise. The pancreas, in response, will secrete insulin to bring blood-sugar levels back to normal. However, when we eat carbohydrates with a high sugar-release potential (*see pp18–21*) they send blood-sugar levels soaring far above normal in a relatively short space of time. This is a state known as hyperglycemia. This triggers the pancreas to release a large amount of insulin to bring blood-sugar levels down to normal. Any excess glucose is stored as glycogen, but once the glycogen stores are full, any remaining glucose is stored as fat.

If excess insulin is produced, it will rapidly drain the glucose from the blood, and this can result in abnormally low blood-sugar. This is a state known as hypoglycemia. The symptoms of hypoglycemia can include chronic fatigue, lack of concentration, intense hunger, and irritability. Those experiencing low blood-sugar levels tend to reach for a sugary snack to feel better. This will cause high blood-sugar levels, which trigger a large production of insulin. This results in hyperglycemia. The vicious cycle (*see chart, p15*) then starts all over again and, in the long term, can lead to poor pancreatic function and chronic insulin overproduction known as hyperinsulinism.

Obesity and hyperinsulinism

What distinguishes an overweight person from a person who is slim is that the latter has a pancreas secreting just the right amount of insulin to bring a raised blood-sugar level down to its normal values. The overweight person does not. Instead of releasing the right amount of insulin, the pancreas will secrete more—sometimes much more—insulin than is required to take sugar present in the blood down to its normal level. This is a metabolic disorder known as hyperinsulinism.

In hyperinsulinism, one's whole metabolism is geared toward producing fat, with a subsequent increase in fat reserves. Insulin also indirectly inhibits the breakdown of fat. Researchers in nutrition have demonstrated that the degree to which people are overweight is directly linked to the severity of their hyperinsulinism. From this we can reasonably conclude that the only real difference between someone who is slim and someone who is overweight is that the overweight person suffers from hyperinsulinism, while the slim person does not.

From my own research into diabetes and the glycemic index (GI), which is a system for measuring the sugar-release potential of carbohydrates (*see pp18–21*), and from my own experience of losing weight by eating low-GI foods, I have concluded that obesity could only be the result of hyperinsulinism. In other words, if you eliminate high-GI carbohydrates from your diet, and replace them with low-GI carbohydrates, it will not only suppress hyperinsulinism, but will also trigger weight loss.

> "if your pancreas is performing under par, so too is your metabolism."

Pancreas health check

Most of us know people who consistently eat high-GI foods and remain slim all their life, despite their bad eating habits. This is because they are blessed with a very healthy pancreas that has not lapsed into hyperinsulinism, regardless of the heavy damage inflicted on it over a long period of time.

This is a dwindling minority of the population, though. If you're reading this book, the chances are that this does not apply to you. It is more likely that you, like the vast majority of others, fall into one of the two following camps.

Poor eating habits?
The first (and more common) pancreatic condition is one that develops over the years. Most of us start off with a healthy pancreas that enables us to stay slim for many years, despite bad eating habits. And then, at the age of about 30 or 35, and certainly by the age of 40, we start to put on weight. In later years, some of us even become obese and diabetic.

The pancreas holds out for several decades, but in the end it gives in to the abuse it has suffered.

An inherited problem?
The other scenario includes those like myself, who arrived on earth with a sub-standard pancreas that was inherited. If your parents are overweight (and therefore hyperinsulinic), your chances of having a frail pancreas are high. If your diet from an early age included high-GI foods, it is almost certain that your pancreas is glucose-sensitive, and therefore unwell. And, as we have seen, if your pancreas is performing under par, so too is your metabolism.

Both of the two scenarios mentioned above result in weight gain, and no low-calorie diets or punishing exercise regime will yield sustainable results. The solution lies in normalizing your pancreas and the way it responds to glucose in the bloodstream by eliminating high-sugar foods.

The Glycemic Index

This is a ranking system that measures how much glucose, or sugar, is absorbed into the bloodstream after eating a carbohydrate. Each carbohydrate is assigned a number on the glycemic index, or GI. The number indicates what proportion of the food's total sugar content is absorbed into the bloodstream. The higher the number, the greater the proportion. For instance, lentils have a low GI because only 25 percent of their sugar content is absorbed.

HOW IS IT MEASURED?

Carbohydrate foods contain energy, but not all of this energy is absorbed during the digestive process. Instead of measuring the calories, or potential energy, present in carbohydrates, scientists began to measure the amount of energy, or sugar, actually absorbed from carbohydrates by the body (known as the sugar-release potential of a carbohydrate). This is done by measuring the level of glucose in the bloodstream after eating a carbohydrate. The glycemic index is based on the glycemic value for glucose, which is arbitrarily set at 100. As you might expect, though, most foods have GI values below this level.

Why carbohydrates?

Carbohydrates are the only group of foods that are made up of sugars, and therefore the glycemic index only measures the GI values of carbohydrates. Fats and proteins contain very little sugar, if any (*see pp22–31*). The impact of fats and proteins on blood-sugar levels is negligible, and therefore the glycemic index does not apply to these foods.

The "bad" carbohydrates

These are carbohydrates that produce a large rise in blood-sugar levels, such as potatoes, white bread, white rice, and other refined foods. They have a high GI value (above 50). The body is suddenly in a state of

"If you are overweight, you are probably addicted to bad carbohydrates."

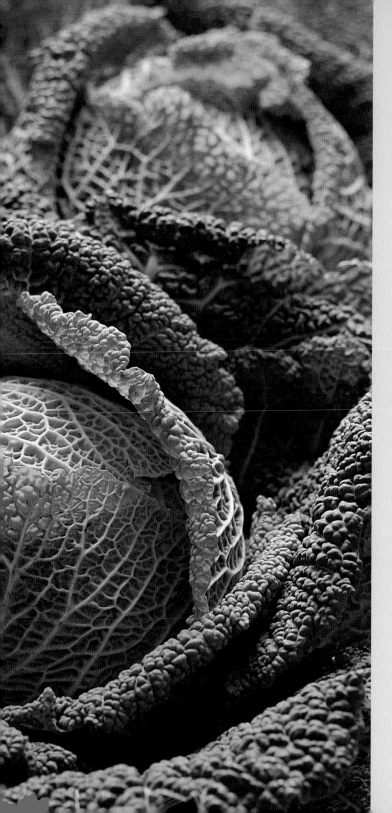

WHAT IS A GOOD GI?

Different sources will tell you different things, but on this diet, I use four distinct bands to classify the GI values of carbohydrates. Low and very low-GI foods are good carbohydrates, while high and very high-GI foods are bad carbohydrates.

• **very low** (GI of 35 or below)
Will result in weight loss.
Foods include vegetables, such as as cabbage, cauliflower, broccoli, zucchini, eggplant, spinach; fruits such as apples, pears, peaches, and cherries; grains and legumes, such as lentils, wild rice, and quinoa.

• **low** (GI of 36–50)
Will prevent weight gain.
Foods include sweet potatoes, brown rice, unrefined Basmati rice, whole wheat pasta, white spaghetti cooked *al dente*, whole wheat bread, kiwi, and grapes.

• **high** (GI of 51–65)
May result in weight gain.
Foods include overcooked white pasta, raisins, corn, refined semolina, and jam made with sugar.

• **very high** (GI above 65)
Will result in weight gain.
Foods include white bread, sticky white rice, rice cakes, white potatoes, popcorn, and cornflakes.

hyperglycemia, where glucose is raised above its normal level. This stimulates the pancreas to secrete excess insulin, which can lead to fat storage and hypoglycemia.

The "good" carbohydrates

Within this diet's framework, good carbohydrates are those foods that yield a small effect on blood-sugar levels. These carbohydrates are assigned relatively low numbers (50 and below) on the glycemic index. They cause only a slight rise in blood sugar, which stimulates a small insulin response from the pancreas. These low-GI foods include many types of fruit and cruciferous vegetables; legumes, such as lentils; and whole grain cereals.

In both the long and short term, low-GI foods will result in the stabilization of blood-sugar levels. This, in turn, will help to desensitize the pancreatic response to glucose. This translates into weight loss or weight maintenance, increased energy, and a general sense of well-being.

Fiber: it's not just sugar content that counts

The amount of sugar a carbohydrate contains is not the only thing that affects its GI value. The GI of a food is also affected by the amount of fiber it contains. This is because fiber reduces the amount of sugar the body can absorb from a carbohydrate. For example, an apple is a carbohydrate that contains sugar in the form of glucose, saccharin, and fructose. It also contains a soluble fruit fiber, known as pectin. This fiber actually reduces the amount of sugar absorbed from the apple by the body. In essence, the apple's fiber content reduces its GI value.

What about refined foods?

The commercial preparation, or refining, of a carbohydrate can raise a carbohydrate's GI value significantly. When foods are refined, they are stripped of nutrients that reduce the amount of sugar that is absorbed into the bloodstream, such as fiber. For example, the GI of brown rice is 50, which makes it a good, low-GI carbohydrate. When brown rice undergoes the refining process it becomes white rice. The new GI of the refined,

"You can reduce the GI of an overcooked starch by letting it cool, and eating it cold."

white rice is 70–20 points higher than it would be for unrefined, brown rice. The reason for this is that when brown rice is refined into white rice, its fiber has been removed, leaving only starch (a form of carbohydrate) behind. The same thing happens when brown whole wheat flour is refined into white flour: all of its fiber is removed, and the GI goes up significantly.

In their new, refined forms, both of these foods now more closely resemble glucose. This allows sugar to pass more easily into the bloodstream, since the body has little work to do in order to break the food down into glucose. Once refined, a good carbohydrate can become a bad one, since most of its complex molecular bonds have been broken in the process.

What about cooking foods?

There are other interesting facts to emerge from the adoption of the glycemic index. Cooking can weaken the molecular bonds in some starchy carbohydrates, yielding a similar effect on GI values as refining a food. Two main offenders are potatoes (*see box, right*) and carrots.

When raw, a carrot is a good carbohydrate with a low GI of about 30. However, when it is cooked, either by boiling, grilling, or steaming, its molecular bonds are broken down, which makes it easier for the body to absorb its sugars and convert it into glucose.

When cooked, the carrot's GI jumps 55 points, from 30 to 85, which makes it a bad carbohydrate. Before you worry too much, I can tell you that this really only affects starchy carbohydrates, such as rice and pasta (*see pp54–57*). The best way to limit the damage is to never overcook these foods, and avoid potatoes and corn completely, particularly when you are on the Rapid Weight Loss Plan.

However, if you do happen to overcook a starch, such as pasta or rice, do not despair. You can reduce the GI of an overcooked starch by letting it cool, and eating it cold. For example, when overcooked spaghetti has been allowed to cool, its GI will actually go down (by up to five points) through a process known as retrogradation. This applies to almost any overcooked starch, excluding carrots, potatoes, and corn.

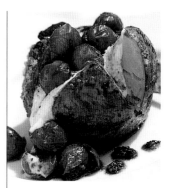

POTATOES

The white potato is a good example of how the cooking process can sometimes make a good carbohydrate into a bad one. When raw, a potato is undoubtedly a good, low GI carbohydrate. Unfortunately, humans cannot digest it when raw. When it is boiled in its skin, however, the GI of a potato shoots up to 65. Mashed potatoes have an even higher GI value of 80. Frying a potato raises its GI even further to 95. The bottom line: completely omit white potatoes from your diet if you want to lose weight.

Proteins

Proteins are the essential building blocks of human body cells, but did you know that they can also facilitate weight loss? This is because the digestion of protein foods, such as meat and fish, involves an increased expenditure of energy. When the body metabolizes protein, it uses up more energy than when it digests fats or carbohydrates. Proteins also leave you feeling fuller for longer, so you will be less inclined to overeat at meals or to snack between them.

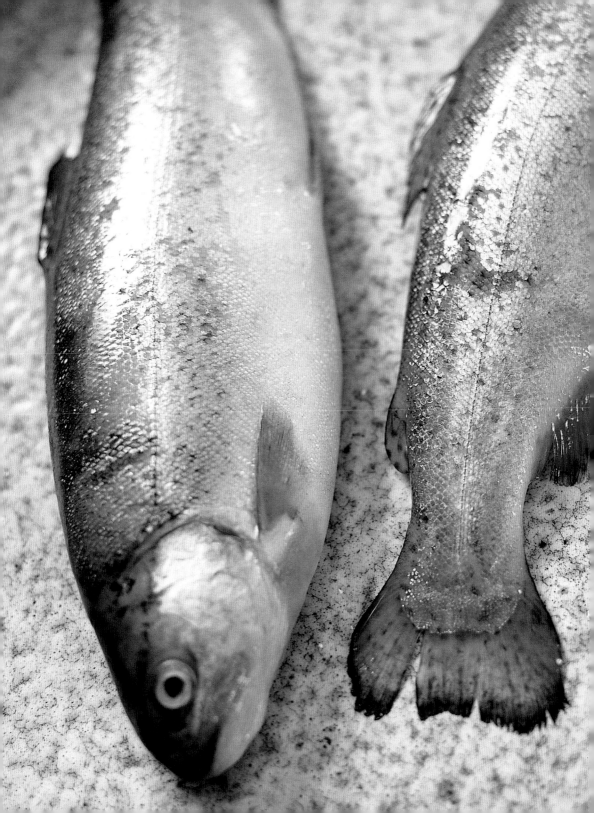

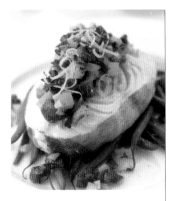

CHOOSE WISELY

Be careful of all of the foods you put into your body, even proteins. Be wary of farmed fish, since they are bred in captivity and fed industrially produced, high-GI foods. In oily fish, this can translate into a reduced quality of omega-3 fatty acids (see p29).

Similarly, you should also beware of processed meats, such as packaged turkey and ham, which are sweetened with glucose. Fresh milk products that still contain milk water (lactoserum or whey) may also yield an increased insulin response, despite their low GI values. This is why it is best to avoid eating too many fresh dairy products. Instead, it is preferable to eat aged or fermented cheese, as French people do.

Montignac on proteins

Proteins are organic substances found in a wide variety of animal and vegetable foods, including foods such as meat, fish, dairy products, and beans. They are essential to the body, and since they contain little, if any, sugar they will not raise your blood-sugar levels, stimulate insulin production, or contribute to weight gain.

THE PROTEIN–WEIGHT LOSS CONNECTION

Protein is essential for good health, and increasing your daily intake can also facilitate weight loss. The reasons for this are twofold. First, the digestion of protein involves an expenditure, since metabolizing protein uses up energy more effectively than metabolizing other foods.

Second, protein leaves you feeling satiated, or fuller, for longer. Feeling satisfied curbs your appetite, which allows you to better control the quality and quantity of the food you eat. It is essential, however, to drink 1.5 to 2 liters of water each day to eliminate body waste, such as urea, uric acid, and lactic acid created by the metabolism of protein.

How much do you need?

For good health, getting an adequate amount of protein in your diet is absolutely essential. For weight maintenance, a good rule of thumb is to eat at least one gram of protein for every 2.2 pounds (1 kilogram) of body weight. This is the amount necessary to compensate for losses caused in the renewal of body cells and to prevent possible wasting of muscle tissue.

This means that if you weigh 154 pounds and you want to maintain your weight you should consume at least 70 grams (2.5 ounces) of protein per day. When your aim is to lose weight, however, you should increase your protein intake to 1.5 grams for every 2.2 pounds (1 kilogram) of body weight, per day. So, this means that to lose weight, you should consume at least 105 grams (4 ounces) of protein per day, though you should see your doctor if you have a chronic health condition before increasing the amount of protein you eat. This ensures that your protein intake exceeds the amount necessary for simple tissue renewal and that it will minimize muscle loss. This will prevent a decrease in your basal metabolic rate (*see pp12–13*), since muscle is actually a metabolically active tissue that burns calories, even while you are resting.

Ideal protein options

The best protein sources for weight loss are foods that are low in fat and high in amino acids (*see box, right*). These include low or nonfat cheeses; eggs; fish; and lean meats, such as skinless chicken or skinless turkey.

Although protein does facilitate weight loss, not all protein is ideal. Some meats, such as beef, pork, and poultry (with the skin on), can be high in saturated fats (*see pp26–31*). When eaten in excess (more than a few times per week), the saturated fats contained in these foods can contribute to cardiovascular disease, or the narrowing of blood vessels. These foods can also trigger weight gain when coated in breadcrumbs or eaten with high-GI carbohydrates, since the insulin these foods elicit can "trap" the fat in the body (*see below*).

How should I prepare my protein?

The goodness of your protein also depends on how the food is prepared. Lean cuts of meat and fish are healthy protein options, but what you do to it does make a difference. For example, almost any type of fish, whether it is tuna, salmon, or cod, is a healthy source of protein when it is grilled, baked, or steamed. The same is true of lean cuts of beef and pork, and skinless poultry.

However, if you take that same piece of protein and coat it with breadcrumbs or flour, it can lead to weight gain. This is not because of the protein itself, but because of the high-GI carbohydrates contained in the breadcrumbs or flour. These foods are high-GI carbohydrates, and they will cause a spike in blood-sugar levels. This, in turn, will trigger the pancreas to release a large amount of insulin.

COMPLETE PROTEINS

Proteins contain large numbers of amino acids, which are used to make cells. Some of these amino acids are made by the body, while others must be obtained from food. There are no vegetable proteins that contain a complete and balanced amount of amino acids and the lack of one essential amino acid can interfere with the absorption of another.

This is why it is essential to eat both animal and vegetable proteins, as a diet consisting of just vegetable proteins will lack some essential amino acids. Vegetarians should include egg and milk protein in their diets, in addition to vegetable proteins such as soy products. Likewise, meat-eaters should incorporate vegetable protein into their diet to avoid nutritional deficiencies.

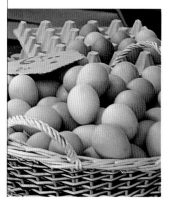

Fats

Fats are complex molecules that store energy for long-term use by the body, but fats don't necessarily make you fat! The key to losing and maintaining weight on this diet is to avoid eating carbohydrates that have high GI values. Since fats contain little sugar (if any), their GI values are often neglible. This means that when fats are eaten on their own, they will not elicit an insulin response and therefore they will not contribute to weight gain.

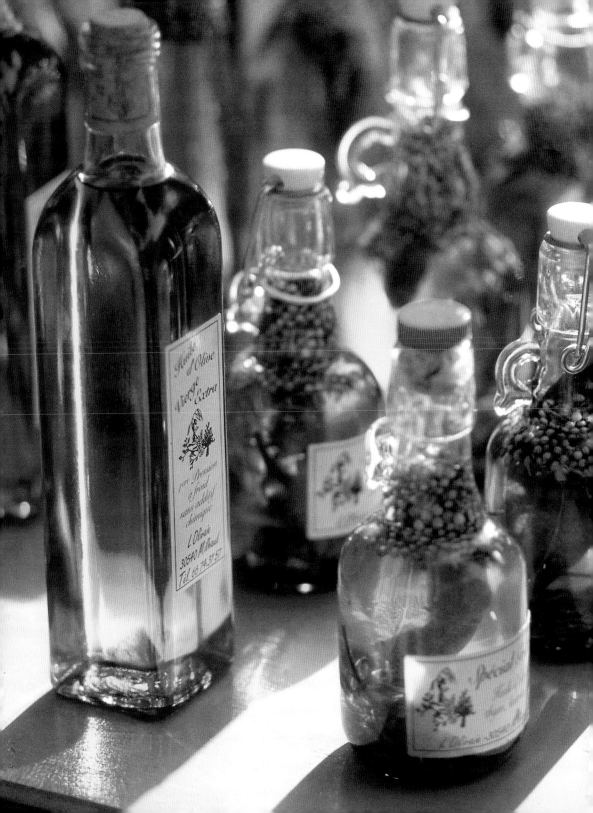

Montignac on fats

Fats, or lipids, are divided into two broad categories, according to their origin. Fats of animal origin are found in meats, fish, butter, cheese, and cream, while fats of vegetable origin include foods such as margarine and olive oil. Rich in a number of vitamins (A, D, E, and K) as well as linoleic acid and linolenic acid (also known as essential fatty acids), fats play a necessary role in a healthy diet when eaten in moderation.

DIFFERENT TYPES OF FATS

Fats can be divided into two main categories: saturated fats and unsaturated fats. Saturated fats are usually derived from animal sources, including meat, butter, cream, and cheese. These fats are solid at room temperature, and they are often thought of as bad fats, since they can increase blood-cholesterol levels and contribute to heart disease.

The other category is unsaturated fats. These fats mostly come from fish and vegetable sources, and are liquid at room temperature. They are considered healthier than saturated fats, since they protect the body against heart disease. Some unsaturated fats actually reduce levels of bad blood cholesterol (also known as low-density lipids, or LDL), which cause narrowing of the arteries, while simultaneously increasing levels of good blood cholesterol (also known as high-density lipids, or HDL). HDL removes built-up cholesterol from the arterial walls, flushing it out of the body. This reduces total blood-cholesterol levels.

Unsaturated fats

There are two main types of unsaturated fats: monounsaturated fats are found in vegetable fats, such as avocados, olive oil, and sunflower oil, and have little effect on blood-cholesterol. Polyunsaturated fats are found in oily fish such as salmon, fresh tuna, and mackerel, and they can actually lower total blood-cholesterol levels (*see above*). Neither of these

"a meal consisting of steak and fries is heresy!"

fats will contribute to weight gain. This is because unsaturated fats, particularly those found in fish, are structurally dissimilar to human fat, and the body must therefore work to convert these types of fat into body fat tissue.

Saturated fats and carbohydrates

As mentioned earlier, eating saturated fats can raise blood-cholesterol levels and contribute to the development and progression of heart disease. But if you eat saturated fat together with a high-GI food, the combination can be doubly dangerous for your health and your waistline. When saturated fats are combined with carbohydrates with a GI above 50, they interfere with the way the body digests fat and, as a result, body fat reserves may be laid down. This is because saturated fats are similar in structure to human fat tissue. The insulin response from the high-GI carbohydrate traps the fat that has been eaten.

So remember, a meal consisting of steak and fries is heresy! Meat, of course, contains unsaturated fat and potatoes are a high-GI carbohydrate. The high levels of insulin circulating in the bloodstream caused by eating the potatoes will ensure that the fat from the steak will be deposited in your body as fatty tissue. The ultimate result will be weight gain. What's more, the weight you gain will be proportional to the quantity of fat consumed with the meal.

Eat fat and stay slim

If you do not have a history of high cholesterol, there is no need to be alarmed about saturated fat. It is bad for your heart, but when eaten in moderation, it will not cause you to gain weight. On this diet, it is perfectly acceptable to eat reasonable amounts of saturated fats, so long as you do not eat them with high-GI carbohydrates (a GI above 50). When eating a meal that contains saturated fats, you must restrict your carbohydrate choices to foods with a GI value of 50 or below. This is because low-GI carbohydrates, including beans and other vegetables, will only stimulate the pancreas to produce a small amount of insulin, which is not enough to trap and store the fat in the body.

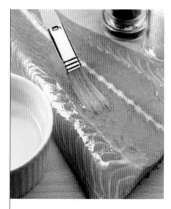

OMEGA-3 FATTY ACIDS

Oily or fatty fish, such as salmon, sardines, herring, and tuna, contains polyunsaturated omega-3 fatty acids, which have various protective and therapeutic properties. Omega-3 fatty acids are particularly good for the heart. I recommend eating as much fatty fish as possible, since it will never contribute to weight gain.

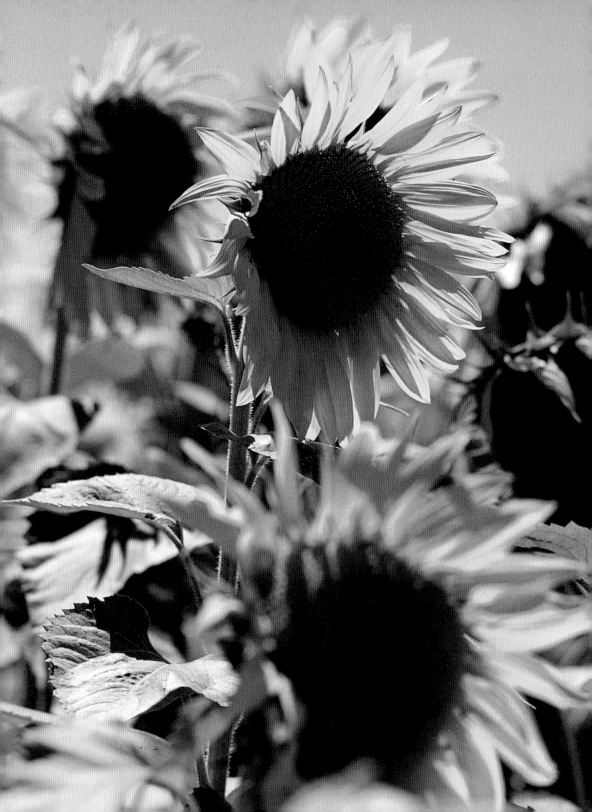

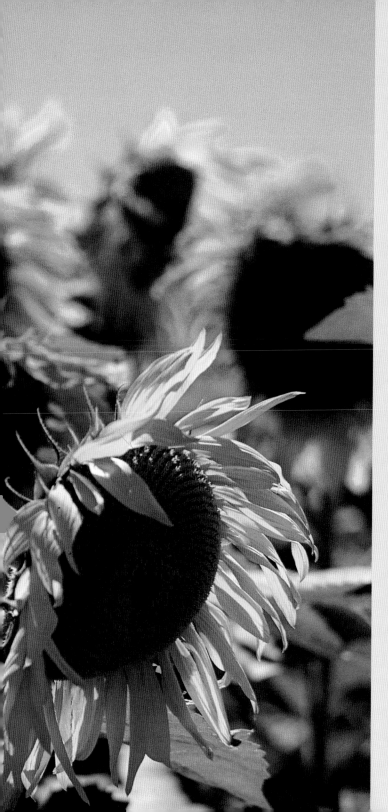

HEALTHY FATS

If you are concerned about heart disease, you should replace saturated fats (found in animal fats, such as butter) in your diet with unsaturated varieties. Unsaturated fats, including oil made from sunflowers, can help protect against cardiovascular disease by increasing your good cholesterol levels (*see pp28–29*), while reducing bad cholesterol.

High levels of triglycerides (the main form of fat in adipose tissue), also known as hypertriglyceridemia, can also contribute to cardiovascular disease. This condition can be caused not only by eating saturated fats, but also by consuming high-GI carbohydrates. So, a diet rich in unsaturated fats and low-GI carbohydrates can significantly reduce triglyceride levels, bad cholesterol levels, and your risk of cardiovascular disease.

Carbohydrates

All sugars and starches are carbohydrates.
After being transformed into glucose, the sugar and starches from the carbohydrates are absorbed into the bloodstream within 30 minutes. However, the amount of glucose released into the bloodstream is determined by the carbohydrate's glycemic index. Any sugar not absorbed after 30 minutes may be excreted, unused by the body. The concept of fast and slow-releasing carbohydrates is a myth.

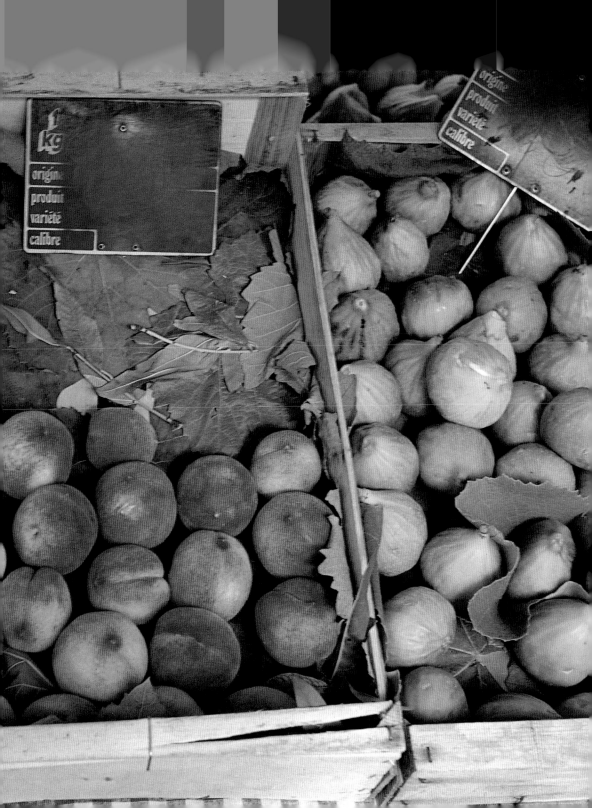

Montignac on carbohydrates

Carbohydrates, also termed sugars, provide the body with its primary source of fuel—glucose. However, eating too many high-GI carbohydrates can lead the pancreas to flood the bloodstream with an excess of glucose, which, in turn, can contribute to weight gain.

TYPES OF CARBOHYDRATES

There are several types of carbohydrates, which are classified according to the complexity of their sugar molecules. Carbohydrates composed of single molecules of sugar are known as monosaccharides. Disaccharides, or carbohydrates containing two molecules of sugar joined together, include sucrose (sugar) and maltose (found in beer). These carbohydrates tend to have high-GI values, and they are referred to as simple sugars.

What about starches?

Starches are known as polysaccharides, which are made up of hundreds of glucose and sugar molecules joined together. They are found in bread, grains, beans, seeds, and in most vegetables. These are known as complex carbohydrates. The GI of a starch is not based strictly on its sugar content, but also on its fiber content (*see box, right*). Refined starches that are low in fiber, such as white bread, have high-GI values and are terrible for your weight. Those that are rich in fiber, including green vegetables, have low-GI values and can be eaten with a minimal risk of weight gain.

The fast/slow sugar myth

For many years, scientists and nutritionists placed carbohydrates into two distinct categories: "quick sugars" and "slow sugars." These terms referred to the speed at which it was thought the body assimilated the sugars.

"the lower the glycemic index of the carbohydrates you eat, the lower your weight will be."

Simple sugars (monosaccharides and disaccharides) were called "quick sugars." People believed that the simple nature of the molecule meant that these sugars were rapidly assimilated by the body after eating them.

Conversely, complex carbohydrates were called "slow sugars," since they contain a chain of sugar molecules which have first to be chemically transformed into simple sugar (glucose) during the course of digestion. This term applied most notably to the starches in whole-grain foods, from which it was thought that glucose was released into the body slowly. This way of classifying carbohydrates is outdated today, since it is based on a mistaken theory.

The new verdict

Recent studies show that the complexity of a carbohydrate's make-up does not determine the speed with which glucose is released into the bloodstream. In other words, the glycemic peak (that is, the point of maximum glucose absorption) is reached at the same rate for any carbohydrate eaten in isolation and on an empty stomach. This occurs about half an hour after ingestion. So, instead of talking about the speed of assimilation, it is more important to consider the effect different carbohydrates have on the blood sugar levels — that is, how much glucose they produce in the bloodstream. Therefore, carbohydrates are now classified according to their potential to raise blood sugar levels, as defined by the GI (*see pp18–21*).

Carbohydrates and your weight

The GI of the foods you eat has a direct correlation to your weight and your health. In other words, the lower the glycemic index of the carbohydrates you eat, the lower your weight will be. High-sugar carbohydrates have a GI of above 50. Moderate-GI foods containing a moderate amount of sugar have values between 35 and 50, and low-sugar foods have relatively low GI values of 35 and below.

Refined carbohydrates, such as white bread, have a simpler structure and release more sugar than unrefined carbohydrates such as whole-grain bread. As a general rule, carbohydrates with simple structures tend

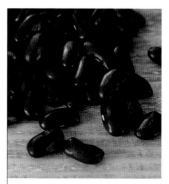

HIGH-FIBER CARBOHYDRATES

Dietary fiber is a substance found mainly in beans, vegetables, fruit, and whole-grain cereals. Although it has no actual calorific value, fiber plays an important role in the body. Fiber keeps waste products such as fecal matter moving through the digestive tract, thereby preventing constipation. It also reduces the body's absorption of fats and certain toxic food additives, such as artificial colorings. Most importantly, though, fiber has a beneficial effect on obesity. A diet rich in fiber can reduce the levels of glucose absorbed and, subsequently, the amount of insulin released into the bloodstream.

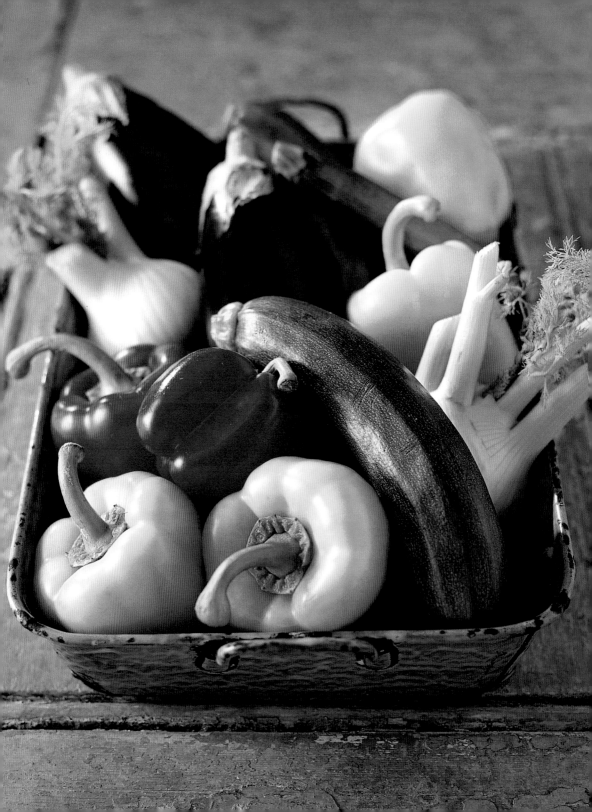

to have higher GI values than those with complex structures. This is because the body has to do very little to convert these "simple" carbohydrates into glucose, which raises blood-sugar levels.

The body has a more difficult time extracting glucose from complex carbohydrates. As stated earlier, the body has a 30-minute window during which it must absorb the glucose from a food. If it has not done so during this period, the sugar is thought to simply be excreted from the body, rather than used.

Carbohydrates and weight loss

To lose weight you must exclude carbohydrates with a GI in excess of 35 for most meals. This rules out foods such as white bread, white rice, and potatoes, not to mention sugary sodas and other sweets, to keep your insulin response as low as possible. This will not only prevent your body from storing fat, but it will also jump-start the process of breaking down fat stores to provide additional energy for the body, as required. It sounds difficult, but this stringent period is just that—a finite period. For weight maintenance, your choice of carbohydrates is broader, and includes foods with a GI of up to 50.

Carbohydrates and general health

It is important to note that the GI of the carbohydrates you eat not only affects your weight, but it can also have an enormous impact on your general health. For example, eating low on the glycemic index may have the added benefit of reducing your total blood cholesterol and triglyceride levels (different forms of fat in the body) if you keep your intake of saturated fats to a minimum as well (see pp26–31).

In addition, eliminating high-GI foods can prevent the onset of type II diabetes, a chronic metabolic disorder. Type II diabetes usually develops over a period of time, and it most commonly affects those who are overweight. Its causes are closely connected to poor glucose tolerance (see pp14–17) and it occurs when the body's cells become resistant to insulin secreted by the pancreas. Adhering to this diet plan can prevent type II diabetes from developing in the first place.

"The countries that have the lowest incidence of cardiovascular disease are those that consume olive oil, fruit, beans, and drink wine."

Left, opposite: eggplant, zucchini, fennel, and peppers have low GI values and are good carbohydrates.

How the diet works

This is not a diet in the traditional sense of the word, since it does not restrict the amount of food you can eat over a short period of time. This diet is a balanced way of eating, based on good food choices. Follow the diet's guidelines on selecting your foods wisely, and you will revitalize your metabolism and shed unwanted weight, permanently.

THE GUIDING PRINCIPLES

There are two main principles that you should remember when following this diet. The first requires you to completely forget about counting calories. The calorific content of food is not important for those who wish to lose weight (*see pp12–13*).

The second guiding principle is that you must choose foods based on their metabolic potential. In other words, choose carbohydrate foods based on the amount of energy, or glucose, that will be absorbed by the body, as expressed by their GI values.

The Golden Rule

For weight loss, the diet's golden rule is based on eating as low on the glycemic index as possible. In other words, choose carbohydrates that have low or very low GI values. If your aim is to lose weight quickly, you should choose carbohydrates with a GI value of 35 or below for most meals (*see pp104–105*). For weight maintenance, or if you choose to lose only a little bit of weight, you may eat carbohydrates with a GI as high as 50, but no higher than this (*see pp152–53*).

For general health, I urge you to choose lean, high-quality proteins. You must also keep your saturated fat intake to a minimum, and choose instead polyunsaturated omega-3 fatty acids (*see pp26–31*), found in fatty fish, such as salmon and mackerel, and monounsaturated fats, such as olive oil and avocados.

"This diet is a balanced way of eating, based on good food choices."

Two plans for two goals

There are two plans in this diet: the Rapid Weight Loss Plan (*see pp44–105*) and the Weight Control Plan (*see pp106–53*). How rigorous you are in adopting a low-GI way of eating is what distinguishes the two plans from one another.

The Rapid Weight Loss Plan is for people who want to lose weight quickly or have a lot of weight to lose. It is naturally a bit more restrictive in terms of the foods you may eat. After you have lost your excess weight and have renormalized your pancreas's response to glucose, you should gradually implement the Weight Control Plan over a period of a couple of months for weight maintenance.

If, however, you are more relaxed about how quickly you wish to lose weight or if you do not have a weight problem, you may skip the Rapid Weight Loss Plan altogether and go straight to the Weight Control Plan. This broader and more permissive eating plan is ideal for those who simply want to eat well, feel terrific, and maintain their current weight.

Where to begin

Before you do anything else, you should set yourself a goal weight. It is important to remember, however, that no two bodies are alike. Some people are more sensitive to glucose than others, and factors such as age, gender, eating habits, and heredity all play a part in determining your weight. These variables make it difficult to determine how much weight you will lose each week.

If you want to lose a lot of weight, I suggest that you begin with the Rapid Weight Loss Plan, which can last from several weeks to several months. If you reach your goal weight in a very short period of time, you may be tempted to stop this plan as soon as you have reached your goal weight. I would advise against this. This is because the aim of the Rapid Weight Loss Plan is not just to lose weight, but also to stabilize the way your pancreas functions and to raise its tolerance threshold to glucose. This normally takes one to two months. If you cut this plan short prematurely, you may have achieved your goal weight, but you also run the risk of failing to give your pancreas time to become healthy again.

A FRESH START

Perhaps you already have a fairly good idea of how much weight you would like to lose. Many people are happy to lose 10 pounds, even though they really need to shed twenty pounds.

Past failures with stop-and-go low-calorie diets may have lowered your expectations. With this diet, however, I would encourage you to be ambitious and set your sights as high as possible.

Good and bad carbohydrates

Since carbohydrates are the only foods that contain sugar, GI values apply only to these foods. Fats and proteins contain very little sugar and therefore their impact on blood sugar levels are negligible (see pp22–31). For the complete chart of carbohydrates, with precise GI values, see pages 240–45.

Good carbohydrates (GI of 50 and below)	Bad carbohydrates (GI over 50)
Freshly squeezed fruit juice (no added sugar)	Beer
Sweet potatoes	White potatoes (baked; fried or french fried; mashed)
Whole wheat or rye bread (made from unrefined flour)	White bread
Spaghetti, whole wheat (cooked al dente)	Ravioli; tortellini; overcooked spaghetti
Unrefined cereals	Refined cereals (e.g. cornflakes)
Wild rice	Semolina
Fructose	Glucose; honey; sugar
Brown rice; unrefined Basmati rice	White rice; puffed rice; rice cakes
Carrots (raw)	Carrots (cooked)
Natural (unflavored) yogurt (sugarfree)	Fruit yogurt (sweetened with sugar)
Peas (dried)	Corn (fresh; steamed; popcorn)
Quinoa	Couscous
Oat cakes (sugarfree)	Crackers (made from refined flour)
Dried fruit (figs; prunes; apricots)	Raisins; sultanas; dried bananas; dried coconut
Beans (haricot; green; flageolet)	Risotto
Chickpeas (garbanzo beans)	Tapioca
Flour, whole wheat (unrefined)	Flour, bread (refined)
Fruit jam and jelly (sugarfree)	Fruit jam and jelly (sweetened with sugar or grape juice)
Dark chocolate (70 percent cocoa)	Milk chocolate
Cruciferous vegetables	Some starchy vegetables (e.g. parsnips; pumpkin; turnips)
Fresh fruits (excluding bananas; melon; watermelon)	Watermelon; melon; bananas

Good and bad fats

This diet advocates choosing good, low-GI carbohydrates. However, it is also important to eat unsaturated fats and limit your consumption of saturated fats (particularly if you have high cholesterol). The fats below marked with a cross are polyunsaturated, and may reduce total cholesterol.

Good fats (unsaturated)	Bad fats (saturated)
Herring+	Butter
Salmon+	Lard
Tuna+	Beef dripping
Mackerel+	Pork dripping
Sardines+	Lamb dripping
Avocados	Fatty cuts of red meat
Olive oil	Poultry skin
Sunflower oil	Pâté
Sunflower seeds	Hard, stick margarine
Walnuts	Hydrogenated oils
Walnut oil	Palm oil
Corn oil	Peanuts
Goose fat	Peanut oil
Macadamia nuts	Coconut
Brazil nuts	Coconut oil
Almonds	Cheese
Flax seeds	Cream
Canola oil	Whole milk
Pumpkin seeds	Full-fat crème fraîche
Pumpkin seed oil	Whole-milk yogurt

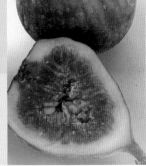

why it works

digested chapter

low-calorie diets can actually slow the rate at which your body burns calories, which will invariably lead to weight gain after the diet has ended.

excess weight is the result of an unwell pancreas that over-responds to glucose in the bloodstream and produces too much insulin, which leads to glucose being stored as fat instead of burned for energy.

the glycemic index is a ranking system that measures the amount of sugar the body will absorb from carbohydrates.

good carbohydrates have a GI value of 50 or below. They will not elicit a large insulin response, or cause you to gain weight.

KEY POINTS TO REMEMBER

_____ **bad carbohydrates** have GI values above 50. They will trigger a large insulin response, which will contribute to weight gain.

_____ **proteins** are the essential building blocks of life, and they can actually facilitate weight loss. They contain a negligible amount of sugar and they are not measured by the glycemic index.

_____ **good fats** are unsaturated and found in oily fish and vegetable oils. Because they are structurally dissimilar to human fat tissue, they are not easily converted to fatty tissue by the body.

_____ **bad fats** are saturated and found in animal products, such as butter. Avoid bad fats, especially when eating a carbohydrate with a GI higher than 50. This food combination can cause you to gain weight.

_____ **a low–GI diet** will help you to control your weight by suppressing hyperglycemia and hyperinsulinism. The lower you eat on the glycemic index, the more weight you will lose.

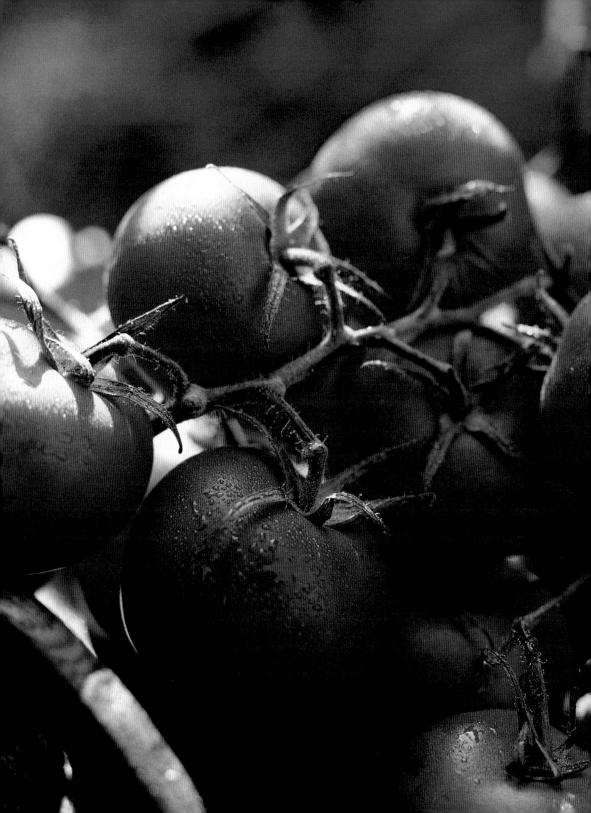

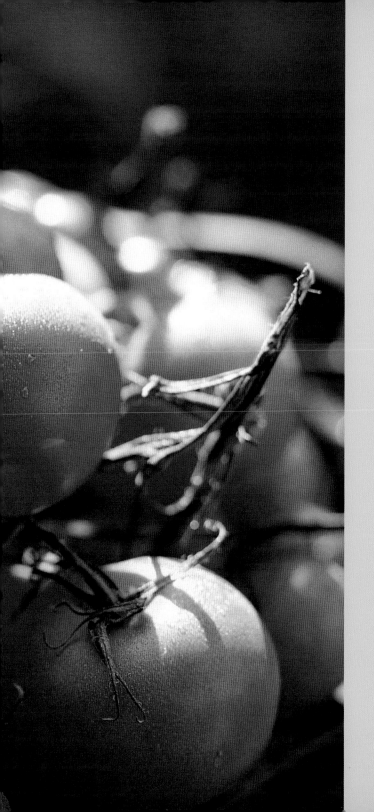

RAPID WEIGHT
LOSS PLAN

In a nutshell

If your goal is to lose weight quickly and permanently, then the Rapid Weight Loss Plan is the right place to start. It will show you how to choose foods that will renormalize your pancreas, boost your metabolism, and trigger fat loss. Before you embark on this plan, however, it is essential that you read all of the preceding pages so that you fully understand the basic principles of the diet.

THE OBJECTIVES

The aims of the Rapid Weight Loss Plan are two-fold, but interconnected. First, to facilitate fast, healthful, and sustainable weight loss. Second, to calm the way in which your pancreas produces insulin and to reduce its sensitivity to glucose. This, in turn, will improve the efficiency of your metabolism, which will allow you to maintain your weight loss.

Weight loss

If you are used to eating a lot of sugar, or are a dessert fanatic, you will probably experience a dramatic weight loss during your first week on the Rapid Weight Loss Plan. This is a normal response, since your body is probably not used to this healthful way of eating. But do not abandon the plan at this point, because in just two days of returning to your old eating habits, you risk regaining the weight it took you a week to lose (*see duration, opposite*). After this initial period, weight loss will occur steadily, but less dramatically than in the first week.

Stabilizing the pancreas

If you are overweight, then it is likely that your pancreas over-responds to bad carbohydrates (such as white bread) by releasing too much insulin in response to the glucose in your bloodstream. At the very least, you will have poor glucose tolerance, and you may even be suffering from

"You may find that you lose your excess weight very quickly."

hyperinsulinism (*see pp14–17*). Both of these conditions are linked to an addiction to high-sugar, high-GI carbohydrates. The amount of insulin your pancreas produces is no longer in the right proportion to the amount of glucose released into your bloodstream after eating a carbohydrate. In short, your pancreas produces too much insulin, which, in turn, leads to weight gain.

Following the rules of the Rapid Weight Loss Plan will help you to normalize your pancreas. This will raise your glucose tolerance threshold so that when you do eat a carbohydrate, your body will respond by releasing an appropriate amount of insulin. This will help you to lose weight and keep it off permanently.

The duration

You may find that you lose your excess weight very quickly and, because of this, you may be tempted to cut short the duration of the Rapid Weight Loss Plan. You must not succumb to this temptation! Remember, the goal of this plan is not only to lose weight quickly, but to make your pancreas function normally so that you can keep the weight off. No matter what your goal is, you must remain on the Rapid Weight Loss Plan for at least a month (and preferably three months) in order to stabilize the metabolic and digestive functions of the body. Sustainable weight loss is not possible without a properly functioning pancreas, and it can take up to three months for this to occur. If you abandon the plan too soon, you may not have given your pancreas sufficient time to recover its equilibrium. If you end the Rapid Weight Loss Plan too soon, your success will be short-lived.

What next?

Now that you have familiarized yourself with the foundations of the diet and the basic objectives of the Rapid Weight Loss Plan, you are probably wondering how to get started. The following section will outline the rules of the Rapid Weight Loss Plan, which will provide you with everything you need to know about using this eating plan for maximum weight loss. Good luck!

OTHER BENEFITS

If you suffer from hypertriglyceridemia or high cholesterol (*see pp30–31*), this diet should have a therapeutic effect on these levels. Studies have shown that a diet laden with high-GI carbohydrates and saturated fats can contribute to these conditions. This diet restricts the consumption of both of these types of foods, while encouraging the intake of heart-healthy, low-GI carbohydrates and unsaturated fats. This approach has been proven to reduce elevated levels of cholesterol and triglycerides.

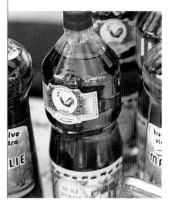

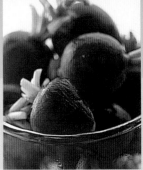

rapid weight loss
the rules

1   **never skip a meal,** particularly lunch. Eat until you are full, and remember that counting calories is a useless exercise. Simply follow the basic principles and eat three balanced meals a day at regular intervals.

2   **there are two breakfast** options. Option 1, the carbohydrate-protein breakfast, can include high-fiber bread, but it must be free from saturated fat. Option 2, the protein-fat breakfast, excludes carbohydrates. Because this meal is high in saturated fat, you should only have it twice a week.

3   **there are two types** of lunch and dinner: Option 1, the protein-fat meal, consists of protein and carbohydrates with a GI of 35 and below. Option 2, the high-fiber carbohydrate meal, contains carbohydrates with a GI as high as 50, but the meal must not include any saturated fat at all.

4   **have up to four** high-fiber carbohydrate meals per week. Meals can contain carbohydrates with a GI up to 50, but they must be low in saturated fat.

5   lunch and dinner

lunch and dinner are very similar, but your dinner should be lighter than your lunch. That is, dinner should contain less fat and meat and more low-GI vegetables.

6   eliminate sugar

eliminate sugar in all its forms. This includes not only obvious sugar sources, such as desserts, but also high-GI carbohydrates, and drinks, soups, jams, and other condiments, which can contain hidden sugar.

7   avoid caffeinated beverages

avoid caffeinated beverages since caffeine triggers the pancreas to secrete insulin. Avoid coffee, sodas, and strong black tea, and drink weak or herbal tea, decaffeinated or Arabica coffee, and water instead.

8   limit alcohol consumption

limit alcohol consumption and never drink it on an empty stomach. One 3.5-fl oz glass of wine or one 3.5-fl oz glass of beer can be drunk with your lunch and dinner, provided you have eaten a protein-fat snack or some of your meal before taking your first sip.

9   avoid eating

avoid eating saturated fats with carbohydrates with a GI above 35. You may have a small amount of monounsaturated fat, such as olive oil, or polyunsaturated fat, found in fatty fish such as salmon. Fish oil will not contribute to weight gain.

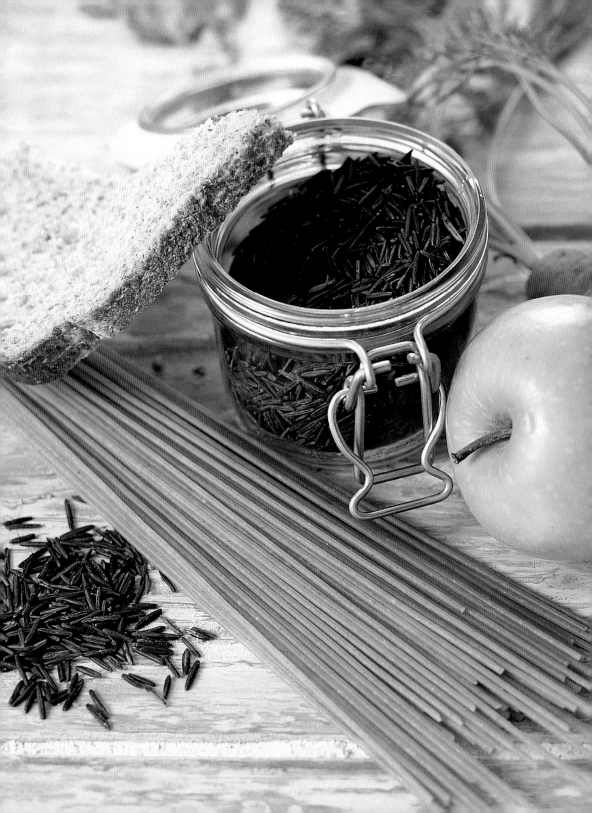

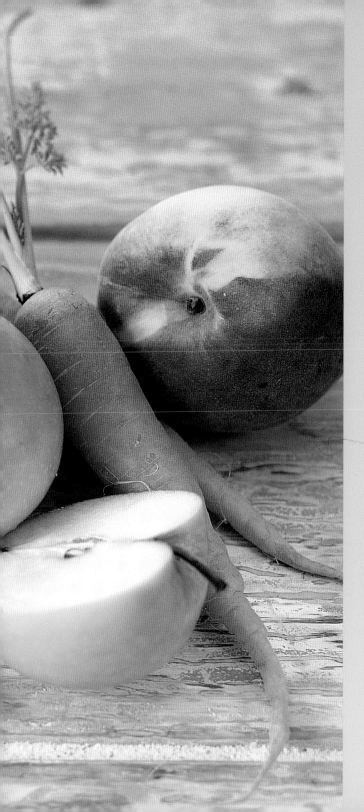

Choose foods wisely

Some seemingly healthy foods can actually have dangerously high GI values. This section will examine a few of the big offenders and show you how to choose these caution foods in their least glycemic forms.

- sugar

- starches

- bread

- pasta

- fruit

- drinks

On sugar

Sugar is a colossus in the world of bad carbohydrates. It should come with a health warning, just like cigarettes, for it can be dangerous when consumed in large quantities. With the amounts that are added to most foods, we might be forgiven for thinking sugar is an indispensable ingredient in our diet. Nothing could be further from the truth!

THE SUGAR EPIDEMIC

Sugar, by which I mean sucrose, or saccharose, including processed sugars such as white, refined sugar and cane sugar, has a high GI of 70. It is one of the most harmful foods you can put in your body. For tens of thousands of years, man lived quite happily without sugar. The largely indiscriminate use of sugar has evolved in less than 200 years—that is, within the space of five or six generations. It is inconceivable that the human body could adapt fast enough to cope with the perpetually high blood-sugar levels associated with such a radical change in diet.

What's more, the situation has deteriorated even further over the last 50 years as other high-GI foods have been added to our diets. As a result, an increasing number of people are finding that their poor pancreases are unprepared and quite incapable of coping with the heavy demands of a modern high-GI diet. This situation has contributed to the escalating proportion of the population who have found themselves battling with obesity.

What about honey?

Honey is sometimes presented as a healthy and acceptable alternative to sugar, since it is a natural sweetener. However, like sugar, honey has a very high GI value, and it will cause your blood sugar levels to soar; it affects your body in almost exactly the same way as table sugar. In other words, honey is simply another form of sugar to be avoided at all costs.

FRUCTOSE

Compared to ordinary sugar or artificial sweeteners, fructose has definite benefits. To start with, it is a natural sugar and therefore avoids the sort of problems posed by artificial sweeteners. It also has a low GI of 20, which will have little effect on the pancreas and its production of insulin. Finally, it has a similar density to sugar, which means it is well-suited for use in baking and cooking. However, it can increase the level of triglycerides (see pp30–31) in some people when used in significant quantities, so people with cholesterol problems should use it in moderation.

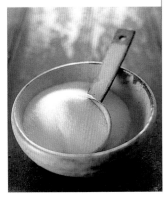

Hidden sugar

There are two types of sugar: the sugar we recognize, and the sugar we don't. The sugar we recognize is the sugar we add to our food and beverages. We have some degree of control over sugar that we've added ourselves, but the sugar we recognize is only half the problem.

The sugar we don't recognize is a far more sinister beast, since it has been added to our food by others without our knowledge. This is hidden sugar, widely used by the food companies and pharmaceuticals industries to give their products bulk and render them palatable for mass consumption. This means that even seemingly benign "foods," such as cough syrups and cough drops, often contain sugar of some kind.

Take a look at almost any food packaging label and you will be amazed at how many commercially prepared foods contain sugar. These hidden sugars can be found under many different names, including sucrose, dextrose, malt, corn syrup, molasses, and honey. Unfortunately, these labels will not always tell you exactly how much sugar has been used, since it is not normally required by law to do so. So, be vigilant when it comes to reading labels, and take nothing for granted.

Maintaining blood sugar

Some may well ask, if we eliminate sugar from our diet completely, how will we be able to maintain minimum sugar levels in our blood? That is a good question and the answer is simple. As has been pointed out in chapter one, the body needs glucose, not sugar, for energy. Fruit, whole foods, beans, and particularly cereals can easily provide the body with all the glucose it needs under normal circumstances. And if there is a temporary lack of carbohydrates to keep the body going (as may happen when the body is engaged in strenuous physical activity), the body is quite capable of drawing on other energy reserves, such as stored fat. So there is no need to eat sugar.

Initially, this may cause problems for people who like to sweeten their food. In which case, I recommend using an artificial sweetener, such as saccharin or aspartame, temporarily until their palates become accustomed to their new regime.

ARTIFICIAL SWEETENERS

Although using artificial sweeteners temporarily can help to wean you off sugar, their prolonged usage could disturb your metabolism in the long term. This is because the body detects sweetness and prepares itself to digest carbohydrates, which then fail to materialize.

Therefore, if you consume a large amount of artificial sweetener during the course of the day, any consumption of genuine carbohydrate in the next 24 hours may result in an excessive spike in your blood sugar level, which is then followed by a hypoglycemic reaction.

Artificial sweeteners exacerbate the hypo- and hyperglycemia cycle (see p15), which, in turn, contributes to intense feelings of hunger and the accumulation of body fat. In short, artificial sweeteners can indirectly contribute to weight gain.

On starches

Starches are complex carbohydrates. Some of them, such as lentils and other legumes, have low GI values and are therefore considered good carbohydrates. However, many starches, including potatoes, white rice, and corn, are bad carbohydrates with high GI values. Eating these starches will prevent you from normalizing your pancreas and losing weight.

THE POTATO

The number one bad starchy food on this diet is the potato. When the potato was brought back from the New World in 1540, the French declined to eat the tuber and gave it to their pigs instead. For two centuries, the French continued to scoff at what they called "the pig tuber". It was not until 1789, when famine raged through the country, that the French finally started to eat potatoes.

Why is it unhealthy?

When raw, the potato is undoubtedly a good food, since it is rich in vitamins and minerals. Unfortunately, it also contains starches that humans are unable to digest. Humans simply lack the necessary enzymes with which pigs are blessed. In order to make potatoes digestible, we must cook them. And although this makes the potato more digestible, it also breaks down its starches, raising its GI value and making it less suitable for our metabolism.

Recent experiments have shown that the potato releases a large amount of glucose when it is digested because of the poor quality of its fiber. When peeled and boiled, a potato has a GI of about 70. Processing the potato (as in instant mashed potatoes) raises the GI to about 80. Fried potatoes, chips, and fries have a GI of 95, and they cannot be ingested without the risk of gaining weight, as the oil used for frying can be laid down as fat reserves.

"When the potato was brought back from the New World, the French declined to eat the tuber and gave it to their pigs instead."

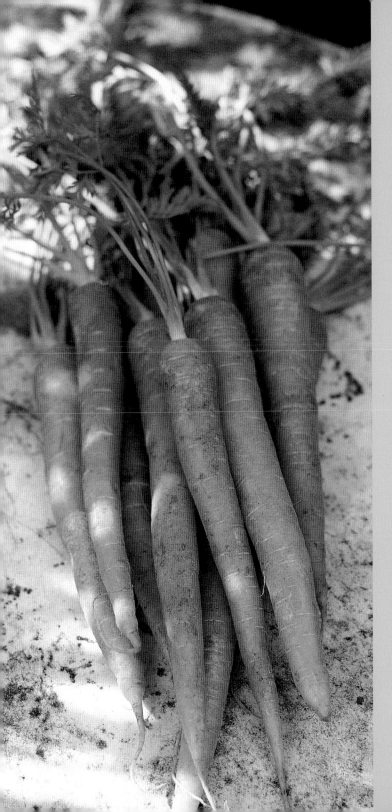

CARROTS

Like potatoes, the starch in carrots is radically affected by heat and the cooking process. Luckily, raw carrots have a low GI of 30, and, unlike raw potatoes, they are digestible by humans. Raw carrots can therefore be eaten freely on the Rapid Weight Loss Plan.

Raw carrots are delicious grated as a side salad, dressed in a vinaigrette. For extra flavor, briefly dry-roast some mustard seeds and sprinkle over.

A carrot only becomes a bad carbohydrate when it is cooked.

Boiling, baking, steaming, or grilling a carrot breaks down its starches, causing the GI to rise dramatically to about 85. Predictably, this makes cooked carrots an unacceptable carbohydrate choice on the Rapid Weight Loss Plan.

However, carrots, raw or cooked, have a low concentration of carbohydrates (*see pp114–15*), which means that on the Weight Control Plan (*see pp106–53*), you can reintroduce cooked carrots into your diet, in moderation.

"White rice, in the form it is eaten in the West, is a highly processed food and a dietary disaster waiting to happen."

On the other hand, when it is boiled in its skin, the GI of a potato can be as low as 65 (although this is still high). Potatoes were usually cooked and eaten this way in the past, together with high-fiber vegetables, which helped to lower the total GI (*see pp112–14*) of the dish by adding fiber.

So, if you want to lose weight on the Rapid Weight Loss Plan, you must avoid potatoes. Forgoing potatoes may be a major sacrifice, but it is worth the price to achieve your goal of a slim and healthy body. Once that goal is achieved, I promise you will have no regrets. If you must have a potato, have a sweet potato instead, since it has a lower GI of 50. On the Rapid Weight Loss Plan, sweet potatoes are acceptable as part of a high-fiber carbohydrate meal, but eat them in the old-fashioned way— boiled or baked with the skin on and served with low-GI vegetables, such as string beans, spinach, cauliflower, or even a salad.

CORN

Maize, also known as corn, is another starchy food that is popular in the Western world. It was grown for thousands of years by the native population of America as part of their staple diet. Still preserved in agricultural museums, the ancient varieties of Indian corn were rich in soluble fiber and had a GI of 35. With the discovery of the new world, Westerners set about growing corn for themselves, and particularly for their livestock. Today's form of corn, however, has a very high GI value and should therefore be avoided on the diet.

Why is it unhealthy?

To increase the amount of corn they could grow, farmers and scientists began a process of selection and hybridization. Within a few decades, the genetic modification of corn caused its GI to almost double to around 65. The starch in today's corn is now so fragile that when it is processed and changed into cornflakes or popcorn, its GI jumps from 65 to 85.

In addition, over-irrigation of modern corn has depleted it of much of its former nutritional content. So, unfortunately, the corn that is available to us today is not the same as it was 500 years ago. It is low in fiber, vitamins, and minerals, but high in bad starch.

As a result, the corn available today causes the pancreas to release a large amount of glucose as it is digested. This, in turn, triggers the pancreas to produce huge amounts of insulin, which can cause pancreatic sensitivity and weight gain. Since they have very high GI values, corn and all corn products, including popcorn and cornflakes, should be omitted from your meals and snacks throughout the diet.

RICE AND OTHER GRAINS

White rice, in the form it is eaten in the West, is a highly processed food and a dietary disaster waiting to happen. It is high in bad starch and very low in fiber and other nutrients. Processing rice, or overcooking it, will raise its GI value even more, and the more glutinous, or sticky, the rice becomes, the higher its GI. For example, pre-cooked rice, or instant rice, has a GI of about 90. Processed products such as rice cakes and puffed rice cakes also have high GI values of roughly 85.

Why is it unhealthy?

White rice is refined to the point that nothing remains of nutritive value except the one thing we could happily do without: starch. Predictably, it is a bad carbohydrate that releases large amounts of glucose into the bloodstream. Ordinary, refined white rice has a very high GI value and should be therefore completely eliminated from the Rapid Weight Loss Plan in the diet.

Conversely, the types of rice eaten in non-Western countries, such as unrefined Basmati and long-grain brown rice, have not been stripped of their fibrous husk, which is a key element in reducing a food's GI value. Therefore, Basmati and long-grain brown rice have a medium GI of about 50 and may be eaten as part of your high-fiber carbohydrate lunches and dinners on the Rapid Weight Loss Plan, and whenever you wish on the Weight Control Plan.

You can also have wild rice (*see right*), which has a very low GI, any time you want. Whatever you do, though, avoid eating refined white rice, puffed rice, and rice cakes at all costs. These high-GI foods will invariably lead to weight gain.

WILD RICE

There are no restrictions on eating wild rice on the diet. Wild rice has a delicious nutty flavor and a low GI value of 35, and you may therefore eat it freely. A little-known fact is that it is in fact an oat, and not a rice at all. Another low-GI carbohydrate to be enjoyed without restrictions is quinoa, a protein-rich, grain-like seed, which also has a low GI of 35.

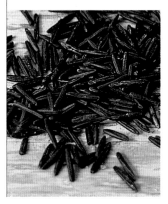

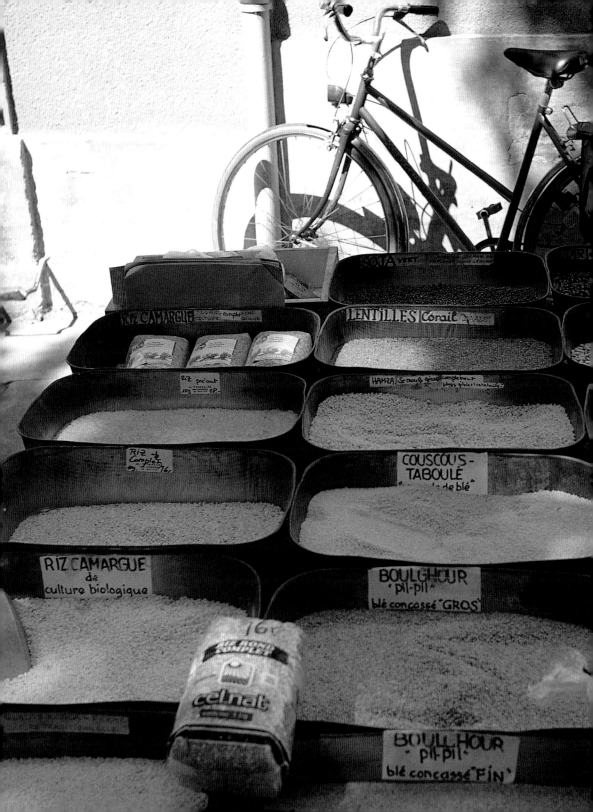

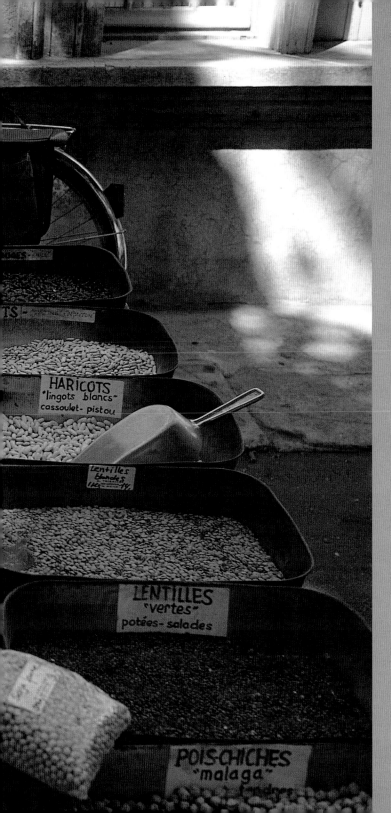

HARICOTS
"lingots blancs"
cassoulet- pistou

Lentilles
blanche S.
...

LENTILLES
"vertes"
potées- salades

POIS-CHICHES
"malaga"

BEANS AND LEGUMES

You might expect me to condemn beans and legumes, given what we know about the potato (*see pp54–56*). Well, you are mistaken! Most beans, including chickpeas, haricot beans, green beans, and split peas, have very low GI values of 35 and below. Lentils have one of the lowest GI of all legumes. Green lentils, for instance, have a GI of 25. Also included here are the distinctive Puy lentils.

These legumes are high in fiber and have very low GI values. They can therefore facilitate weight loss, and are categorized as good carbohydrates. They can be eaten freely at any meal—though without any fat such as butter—on the Rapid Weight Loss Plan. Kidney beans have a slightly higher GI value of 35, and they should therefore only be eaten as part of your high-fiber carbohydrate meals while on the Rapid Weight Loss Plan.

rapid weight loss

cooking starches

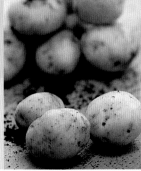

when a potato is peeled and boiled, the GI increases from 65 to 70. When potatoes are processed into instant mashed potatoes, their GI rises by as much as 15 points, from 65 to 80.

french fries or potato chips have a GI value as high as 95 and they cannot be ingested without the risk of gaining weight. This is because the oil used for frying can be laid down as fat reserves.

overcooking rice raises its GI value. The more glutinous, or sticky, the rice is, the higher its GI will be. Pre-cooked rice has a very high GI of 90. Processing rice to make products such as rice cakes and puffed rice gives these foods a high GI value of 85.

——————————— overcooking pasta will increase its GI value. The longer it cooks in the pot, the higher the GI will rise, since more of its starch will gelatinize, and become digestible.

——————— cooking pasta *al dente* keeps its GI as low as possible. Eating pasta cold will cause its GI to go down by a further five points through a cooling process known as retrogradation.

——————————— cooking carrots causes their GI value to rise sharply from 30 to 85, which makes this otherwise good carbohydrate a bad one.

——————— toasting bread may bring down the GI of a piece of bread by several points through a process known as retrogression.

——————————— when corn is heated to produce popcorn, or processed to make cornflakes, its GI increases appreciably, jumping from 65 to 85.

Q&A

Can I eat bread?

Bread could easily have been the subject of a whole chapter. When eaten in moderation, "good" bread, which is rich in fiber, is not fattening. Unfortunately, these days it is a rare commodity. There is plenty of bread around, of course, but most of it is a parody of the real thing, and therefore potentially fattening.

Q How can bread be fattening?

Some breads (but not all) have GI values as high as sugar. Predictably, because your pancreas does not differentiate between foods, it will react to bread or sugar in exactly the same way—that is, by releasing a large amount of insulin to bring down blood-sugar levels. And, as you know, it is this surge in insulin that gives rise to fat storage and weight gain.

Q What kind of bread should I avoid?

White bread, which is made from refined flour, is almost totally devoid of all those elements necessary to feed a healthy metabolism, such as fiber, vitamins, and minerals. Nutritionally, its only contribution to the body is energy in the form of starch. From the digestive point of view, it can only give rise to problems, since it lacks the fiber necessary for good digestion. It is worth remembering that the whiter the bread, the more it should be considered a bad carbohydrate, since the whiteness of color indicates the amount of refining that has taken place.

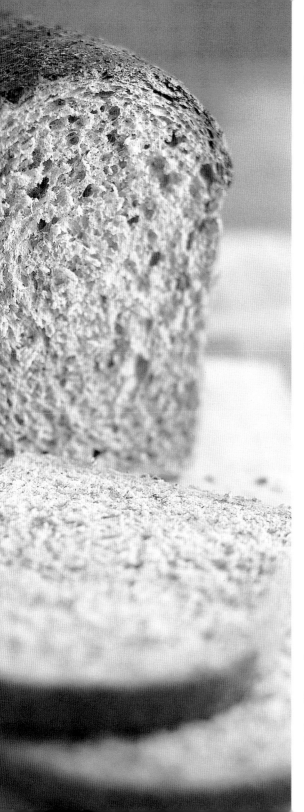

Q What kind of bread can I eat?

High-fiber breads, such as rye, whole wheat bread, or bread made with unrefined organic flour, have the lowest GI values, which range from 40 to 50. Their relatively low GI values have little impact on blood-sugar levels, and so are less "fattening" than refined white bread. As a general rule, the softer and squishier the bread, the higher its GI will probably be.

Q When can I eat bread?

Bread (even good varieties) should only be eaten for breakfast, as part of the carbohydrate-protein breakfast option. This is because even good bread is high in starch, and has a GI value higher than 35. When you start applying the diet's principles, you must be wary of increasing the overall GI of your meal more than necessary in order to keep the level of insulin in your body as low as possible.

"There is plenty of bread around, but most of it is a parody of the real thing."

Can I eat pasta?

You probably expect me to tell you that pasta should be omitted from your diet. In fact, I'll say the opposite: not all pasta is bad. While some pastas have high GI values and should be avoided, other kinds, when cooked in the right way, have relatively low GI values. They can even facilitate weight loss, and are therefore acceptable on the Rapid Weight Loss Plan.

Q Can I eat pasta?

Yes, but the type of wheat used to make your pasta does matter. If you want to eat white pasta, it should always be a pastified variety (*see opposite*) made from hard wheat, and not from soft wheat. Hard-wheat pasta contains more protein and fiber than soft-wheat varieties, and this lowers its GI value. If you are not sure what type of wheat has been used, it's best to avoid white pasta, and eat whole wheat pasta instead. Whole wheat pasta has a higher fiber content than white pasta, which gives it a low GI of 40. Although it is five points higher than the recommended GI of 35, you may eat whole wheat pasta in moderation on the Rapid Weight Loss Plan.

Q When and how often can I eat it?

While following the Rapid Weight Loss Plan, you can eat the recommended types of pasta (*see above*) up to four times per week as part of your three to four weekly high-fiber carbohydrate meals. You should space these meals out over the course of a week; for example, don't have pasta for lunch and dinner on the same day.

Q What is pastification?

Pastification is a mechanical process in which pasta dough is fed through small holes at a very high pressure. This gives the pasta a protective film, which limits the amount of starch gelatinization that can take place during the cooking process. This film lowers the pasta's GI value by about five points, thereby limiting the amount of glucose released into the bloodstream. The most common pastified pastas are spaghetti, linguini, and vermicelli.

Q Does it matter how I cook it?

Whatever pasta you choose, cook it *al dente*, or as firm as possible, since overcooking pasta makes more of its starch digestible, which will increase its GI value. If you accidentally overcook your pasta, you can limit the damage by eating it cold, because the GI goes down through retrogradation, or the cooling process. So, always choose pastified pastas (spaghetti is best) made from a high-fiber flour, and eat it *al dente*.

Q Which pasta has the lowest GI?

Chinese vermicelli, which is really more of a noodle than a pasta, is a different ball game altogether, even though it was the original inspiration for spaghetti. It is different because Chinese vermicelli is not made from wheat flour, like most pastas, but from soy flour. This gives it a very low GI of 22. Since it is also pastified, you can eat as much Chinese vermicelli as you like on the diet. This means that you can include Chinese vermicelli in any of your main meals, regardless of whether they are protein-fat meals or high-fiber carbohydrate meals.

"Chinese vermicelli is a different ball game altogether."

On fruit

Fruit is often a contentious issue when it comes to diets, and were I so foolish as to suggest that you should exclude fruit from your diet, a large number of you would shut the book at this point and read no further. So I will reassure you right away: the diet will not exclude fruit at any point. In most cultures, fruit is a symbol associated with life, health, and vitality—and for good reason. Most fruits are not only delicious, but they are also good for you.

FRUIT AND GI

Fruit contains carbohydrates, such as glucose, saccharin, and, above all, fructose. This means that it is important to be vigilant about the GI—values of fruit. While it's hard to actually gain weight from eating fruit, to trigger fat loss, you must limit your fruit selection to those that have a GI of 35 or below on the Rapid Weight Loss Plan. Luckily, fruit also contains a soluble fiber known as pectin, which lowers the GI by reducing the amount of sugar absorbed by the body.

To peel or not to peel?

Since much of the fiber of a fruit is contained in the skin, peeled fruits tend to have higher GI values than those that are eaten with the skin on. In addition, it is there, close to the surface, that you will find the greatest concentration of vitamins. It is therefore very important to eat the whole fruit, including the skin, in order to keep the GI low and thus help you lose weight more easily.

Fruit won't make you fat

The muscles in the body can easily use the energy available from fruit. Fruit sugar is converted to glycogen and stored in the muscles rather than being turned into body fat. This is why some dried fruits, such as dried

"To trigger fat loss, you must limit your fruit selection to those that have a GI of 35 or below."

figs, can also be considered good, high-fiber fruit options, despite the fact that they have a GI of 40. Some of the best fruit options for rapid weight loss, however, include apples and prunes, which are both high in pectin and have an acceptably low GI value of below 35. (*For more fruit options on the Rapid Weight Loss Plan, see pp68–69.*)

That said, it is best to avoid high-GI fruits, such as bananas, raisins, sultanas, kiwi, watermelon, melon, and grapes while on the Rapid Weight Loss Plan. Their GI values greatly exceed 35, and they may prevent you from losing weight.

Fruit juices

With the exception of lemon juice, which is very low in sugar, it is best to exclude fruit juice from your diet on the Rapid Weight Loss Plan and eat fresh fruit instead. Freshly squeezed fruit juice passes through the body quickly, just as fresh fruit does. However, fruit juice has a higher GI value than whole fruit, since the juicing process strips it of most of its fiber.

Commercial fruit juices, even those labelled "pure fruit," with no added sugar, should be consumed even less often than freshly squeezed juices. Their vitamin and fiber content is lower than that of freshly squeezed fruit, and they normally contain high levels of acid, which is bad for digestion.

Fruit and indigestion

If you suffer from digestive problems, you should eat fresh fruit on an empty stomach only. Contrary to what many believe, this has nothing to do with weight loss, but is rather to help ease digestion. To ensure that your stomach is truly empty, you should only consume fruit three hours after a meal, or at least 20 minutes before a meal.

For some people, eating fruit during or directly after a meal may cause bloating and indigestion, since the fruit can get "trapped" in the stomach, where the heat and humidity cause it to ferment. Luckily, this does not apply to all fruits and there are some exceptions to the rule (*see right*). If you do not suffer from digestive problems, feel free to eat any fresh fruit with a GI value of 35 or below with your meal, or directly following it.

FRIENDLY FRUITS

If you are prone to indigestion (*see left, below*), it is best to eat fruit on an empty stomach. However, every rule has its exception, and there are some fruits that will not cause indigestion. Strawberries, raspberries, blackberries, currants, and lemons can all be eaten during or directly after your meal. They contain so little sugar that they are unlikely to ferment in the gut and cause indigestion. Cooked fruits can be eaten, too, because the cooking process deactivates the enzymes that cause fruits to ferment.

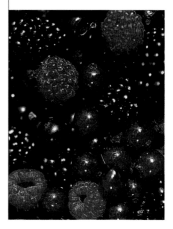

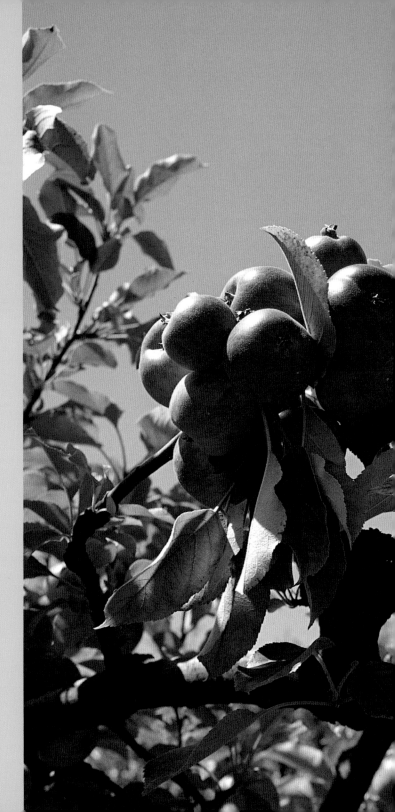

WHAT CAN I EAT?

Apples are one of the best fruits to choose on the Rapid Weight Loss Plan. They are high in vitamins and fiber and have a very low GI. Have them with your breakfast, or on their own for dessert or a snack.

Other fruits that are acceptable for the Rapid Weight Loss Plan include:

- **blackberries**
- **cherries**
- **dried apples**
- **dried apricots**
- **dried figs**
- **fresh apricots**
- **fresh figs**
- **grapefruit**
- **oranges**
- **peaches**
- **pears**
- **plums**
- **prunes**
- **raspberries**
- **strawberries**

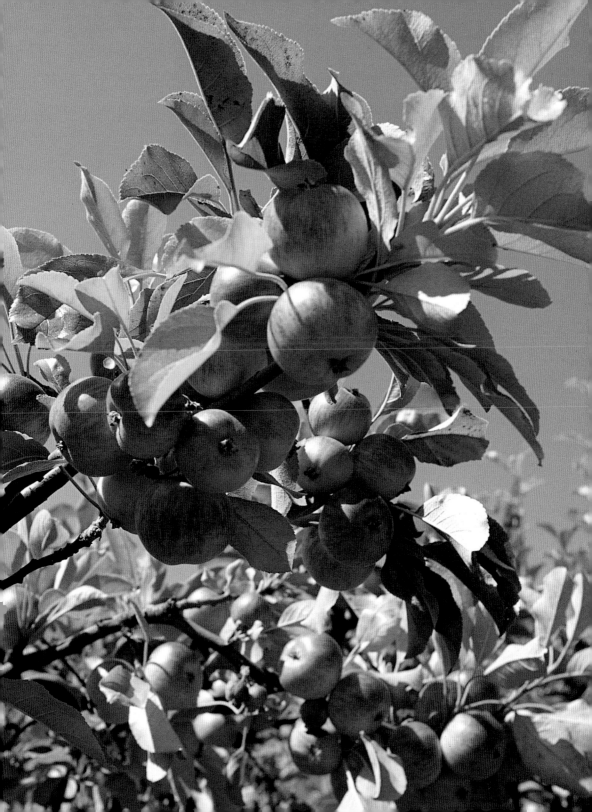

On drinks

What you drink is almost as important as what you eat. Avoid beverages such as fizzy soft drinks, fruit juices, coffee, strong black tea, and whole milk, since they all contain ingredients that may sabotage your new eating regime. Instead, retrain your palette to appreciate the more delicate flavors of still or sparkling mineral water with a twist of fresh lemon or lime.

TEA

Strong black tea can be as bad for your waistline as coffee, since it also contains a lot of caffeine. A better choice would be herbal or fruit teas, such as peppermint or lemon. They are almost always naturally decaffeinated, or contain negligible amounts of caffeine. However, if you can't imagine life without black tea, weak tea can be a good, low-caffeine compromise.

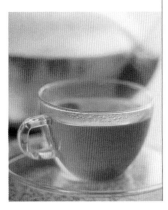

MILK

Whole milk is a complex food, consisting of proteins, carbohydrates (lactose, or milk sugars), and saturated fats. This combination of protein, milk sugar, and saturated fat may encourage weight gain by trapping the saturated fat in the body as fatty tissue (*see pp28–29*).

It is therefore preferable to drink skim milk or if you wish, skim, powdered milk; you can also add skim milk to your tea and coffee. I find that if you use more powdered milk than is recommended, you can produce a thick, smooth liquid that is rich in proteins and can help you to lose weight. (*For more on milk, see pp126–27.*)

COFFEE

Avoid infused coffee, which is made with boiling water and then filtered. It is a wolf in sheep's clothing, since, although it seems light and mild, it contains a lot of caffeine – more than strong espresso. Although coffee is not a carbohydrate, the caffeine it contains stimulates the pancreas to secrete a small amount of insulin. This is why I would advise excluding regular coffee from your regime on the Rapid Weight Loss Plan, and replace it with decaffeinated coffee or herbal tea.

If you feel that you cannot completely eliminate coffee with caffeine from your diet, you can drink pure Arabica coffee. This type of coffee tastes just like regular coffee, but it may contain less caffeine, and it will therefore have less of an impact on your pancreas.

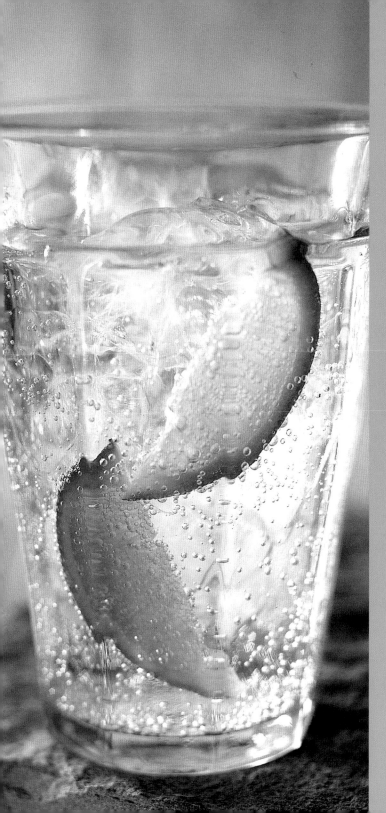

CARBONATED DRINKS

Choose sparkling mineral water with a twist of lemon or lime over colas and other soft drinks. Carbonated soft drinks are usually based on synthetic fruit and plant extracts and have two major flaws: they contain too much sugar and too much caffeine.

Even sugar-free soft drinks can cause an increase in blood sugar levels, since they contain caffeine and artificial sweeteners such as aspartame, both of which trick the pancreas into thinking it is getting sugar (*see pp52–53*).

Carbonated soft drinks also contain artificial gases that give rise to gas and bloating. The worst offenders among these types of drinks are colas, but artificially flavored fruit drinks are nearly as bad. In short, they should be excluded from your diet completely.

Q&A

Can I drink alcohol?

From wine to beer to champagne, alcohol plays an important part in our lives, but when drunk to excess it can lead to weight gain. The diet will show you how to indulge in your favorite beverages without disrupting your metabolism and gaining weight. As long as your consumption of these drinks is reasonable, they should have no effect on your waistline.

Q How does alcohol cause weight gain?

You should not drink alcohol before a meal. If you do, you will not lose weight. This is because alcohol provides energy that is easily used by the body. When you drink alcohol on an empty stomach, the body does not use its fat reserves as a source of energy—it uses the alcohol instead. In this way, alcohol prevents the body losing weight. But this happens only when the stomach is empty. The presence of food in the stomach prevents the alcohol from being immediately released into the bloodstream and speeding up the fat storage process.

Q What should I eat before drinking?

When the stomach is already full, particularly with fats and proteins in the form of meat, fish, and cheese, alcohol is metabolized far less rapidly. Two or three cubes of cheese and a slice of dried sausage, each about the size of a dice, will be sufficient to line the stomach and slow down the rate at which alcohol is absorbed into the bloodstream, thereby preventing a spike in blood-sugar levels.

Q Can I drink wine and champagne?

Yes. One 3.5-fl oz glass of wine or champagne, drunk towards the end of your main meals, will have no adverse effect. Red wine is preferable to white wine since it is rich in antioxidants (*see pp130–31*). Your wine, whether red or white, should be dry and free from additives and preservatives. If these conditions cannot be met, then it is best to drink organic wine or refrain from drinking wine altogether on the Rapid Weight Loss Plan. These drinks won't trigger any insulin response, so you can have up to two small glasses per day on the Rapid Weight Loss Plan. However, you must always eat a small protein-fat snack before taking your first sip.

Q Can I drink apéritifs?

No! Apéritifs must be avoided on this plan. By definition, these are drinks consumed before eating, and this can wreak havoc on your metabolism. Spirits, such as vodka, gin, and whisky, have a very high alcohol content, which will disrupt the metabolism, preventing weight loss and contributing to weight gain. Whenever possible, have a non-alcoholic beverage, such as tomato juice, instead.

Q What about beer?

Beer should be drunk in great moderation, since it not only contains alcohol, but also maltose, a carbohydrate with a very high GI of 110. When beer is drunk between meals, or without eating a protein-fat snack first, it causes weight gain, particularly around the abdomen. If you cannot bear to abstain from drinking beer, you can consume one 3.5-fl oz glass towards the end of each main meal (i.e. lunch and dinner) per day. That said, your attempts at losing weight will be far more successful if you can totally abstain from drinking beer on the Rapid Weight Loss Plan.

rapid weight loss

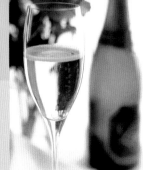

digested chapter

renormalize the way your pancreas responds to glucose in the bloodstream, and you will begin to lose weight. You must stay on this plan for at least three months, even if you lose weight rapidly.

avoid sugar in all its forms. Get in the habit of reading labels, since many seemingly innocuous foods contain hidden sugar.

choose good starches that have a GI of 50 or below. These foods include raw carrots, brown rice, unrefined Basmati rice, wild rice, spaghetti, quinoa, and most legumes, particularly lentils and chickpeas.

avoid bad starches that have a GI over 50. These include white potatoes, white bread, corn, and white, refined rice.

cooking can increase the GI of some carbohydrates by breaking down molecular bonds, which makes more starch digestible. Most notably, this affects carrots, rice, pasta, and potatoes.

eat good bread for breakfast at least five days per week as part of the carbohydrate-protein option. Always choose high-fiber, whole wheat or rye bread, and never eat it with saturated fats.

eat spaghetti, but always cook it al dente. Pastified pastas, such as spaghetti, made from hard-wheat or whole wheat flour have an acceptably low GI value of 40 (or 35 when allowed to cool).

avoid caffeinated drinks, such as coffee, strong tea, and soft drinks, since caffeine stimulates the pancreas to produce insulin.

limit your alcohol intake to no more than two 3.5-fl oz glasses of wine, or 7-fl oz of beer, per day. Never drink alcohol on an empty stomach.

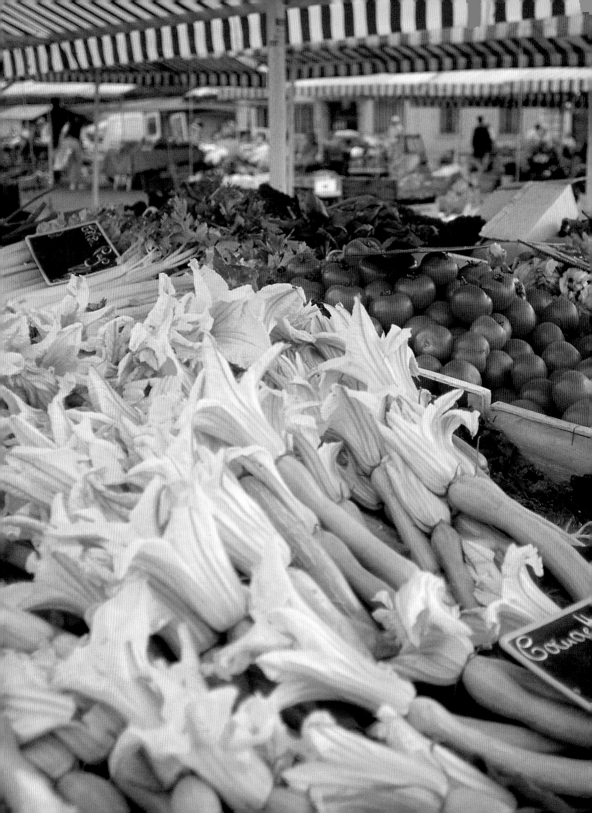

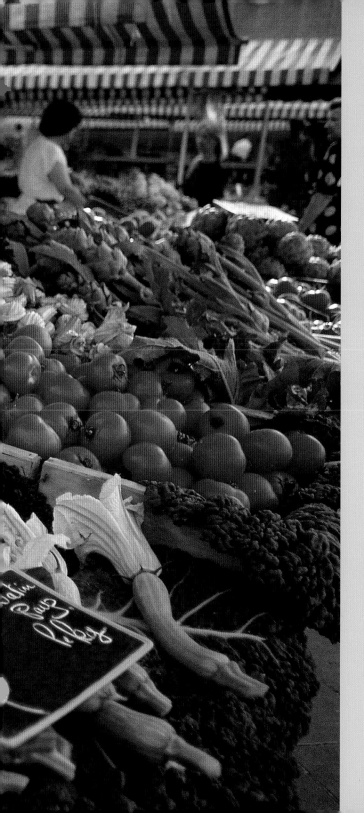

RAPID WEIGHT LOSS: MEAL OPTIONS

Breakfast the Montignac way

There are two types of breakfast you can enjoy on the diet. Option 1 is a carbohydrate–protein meal (*see pp80–81*) and Option 2 is a protein-fat meal (*see pp82–83*). The first option is rich in low-GI carbohydrates and it is the type of breakfast you should have most often—at least five days per week. The second, called the protein-fat option, is high in both protein and fat, and low in carbohydrates. Since it contains saturated fats, this breakfast is less healthy than Option 1, and should be eaten no more than twice per week.

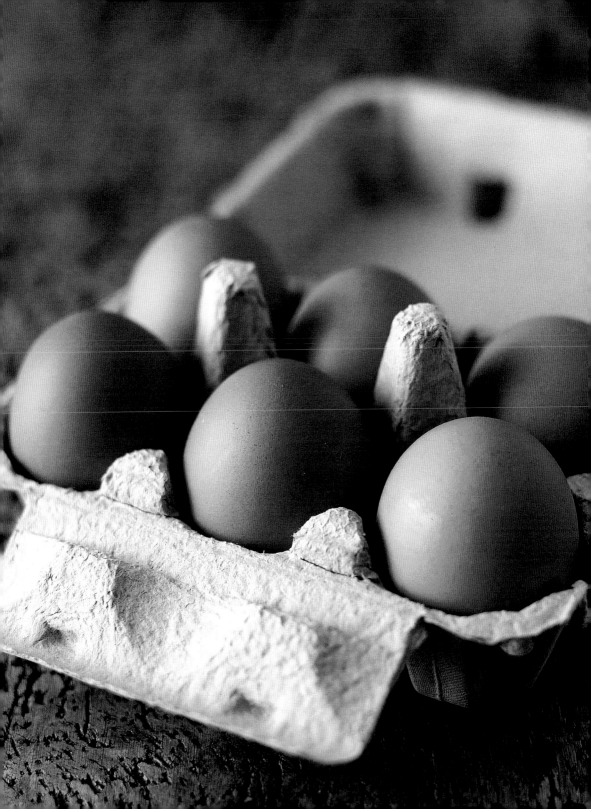

Option 1
carbohydrate-protein breakfast

This breakfast option is a staple meal on the diet and should be eaten on most mornings (at least five times per week). It consists of little or no fat, a low or nonfat protein, and a low-GI carbohydrate. This meal is unique on this plan in that it allows you to have bread. In fact, you can eat as much whole wheat bread as you like with this breakfast, so long as the rest of the breakfast does not contain any fat.

CARBOHYDRATE ELEMENT

The low-GI carbohydrate food is an integral part of this breakfast. You could choose whole wheat or rye toast, since these breads have moderately low GI values. On the Rapid Weight Loss Plan, the only time bread is acceptable is in the morning because your blood sugar level is low upon waking, and your body is unlikely to produce an excess of glucose in response to the bread.

Other carbohydrate options include sugarfree rice cakes or sugarfree whole grain cereal, such as organic oat clusters, mixed oat flakes, or sugarfree muesli. Corn or rice-based cereals should be avoided, since they have high GI values. Eat as much as you like, but make sure that your carbohydrate is rich in fiber and contains no added fat or sugar.

PROTEIN ELEMENT

Your protein element must be very low in saturated fat. Nonfat, soft white cheese, such as nonfat cream cheese, is an ideal protein component since it is rich in protein, free from fats, and low in carbohydrates. Skim milk, nonfat cottage cheese, or nonfat natural yogurt are also good, fat-free protein options. If you like, you can mix some sugarfree fruit jam with your yogurt or cream cheese, or alternatively, you can spread it on your toast or rice cakes.

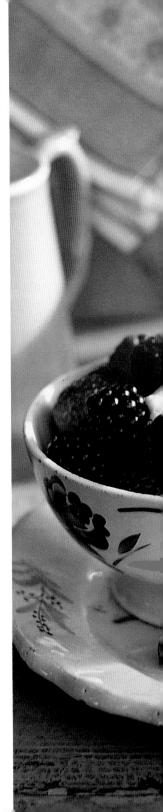

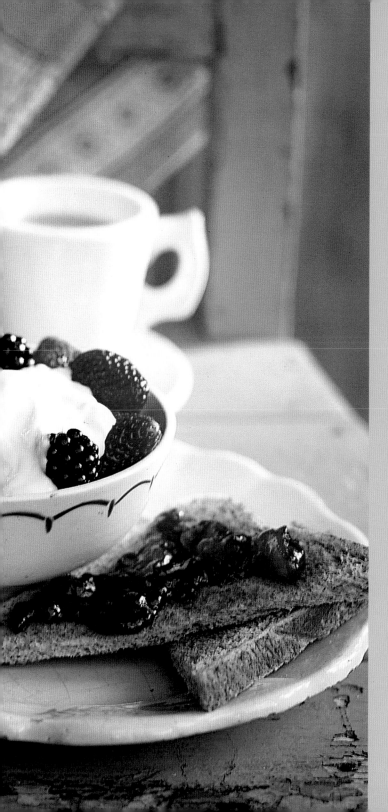

WHAT CAN I EAT?

The breakfast to the left is a
well-balanced carbohydrate-protein
breakfast, which includes whole
wheat toast spread with sugarfree
jam, low-fat natural yogurt with
berries, and a cup of decaffeinated
coffee. To create a different
breakfast, try combining any of the
following elements.

For your carbohydrate
element, choose from the following:
- rye bread
- bread made with unrefined
  organic flour
- sugarfree rice cakes
- sugarfree whole grain cereal

For your protein element,
choose from the following:
- nonfat cream cheese
- nonfat cheese
- nonfat cottage cheese
- nonfat natural yogurt
- skim milk

To drink, choose one of the
following:
- decaffeinated coffee
- pure Arabica coffee
- herbal or fruit tea

Extras can include:
- sugarfree jam or jelly
- fruits with a sub-35 GI value
- fructose or an artificial sweetener

Option 2
protein-fat breakfast

Option 2 is a good breakfast for when good carbohydrates, such as whole grain bread, are unavailable. It contains protein and saturated fat, and it excludes carbohydrates with a GI above 35. This is because these carbohydrates will stimulate the pancreas to produce insulin, which will trap the meal's fat in the body as stored fat. Because of its high saturated fat content, this meal should be eaten no more than twice a week.

PROTEIN ELEMENT

This meal should consist of protein in the form of ham, fish, cheese, or eggs any style. A typical example of this breakfast might be an omelette made with gruyère cheese, served with bacon. It is essential, however, that this meal be completely free from carbohydrates with a GI above 35. This ensures that insulin levels in the blood are kept to a minimum, so that the body will not store the fat you've just eaten. In other words, you should never eat bread, toast, or cereal with this breakfast option, though very low GI vegetables are fine.

FAT ELEMENT

You can prepare this meal using oil or butter and add flavor to your breakfast in the form of fat, such as bacon. These foods are high in saturated fat, and are therefore categorized as the fat component of your breakfast. It is worth mentioning that many of the recommended Option 2 foods are considered complex foods, meaning some of the foods categorized as fat elements contain protein, while some of the protein elements contain fat. Regardless, you may eat as much as you like of any of these foods, so long as your breakfast does not contain carbohydrates with a GI above 35. Balance this meal by selecting foods for lunch and dinner that are high in low-GI carbohydrates and low in saturated fats.

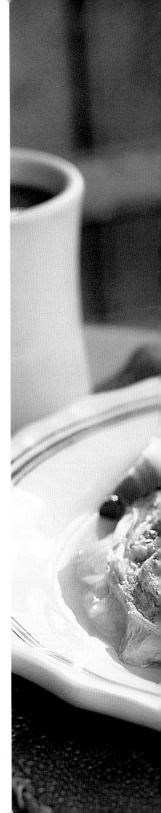

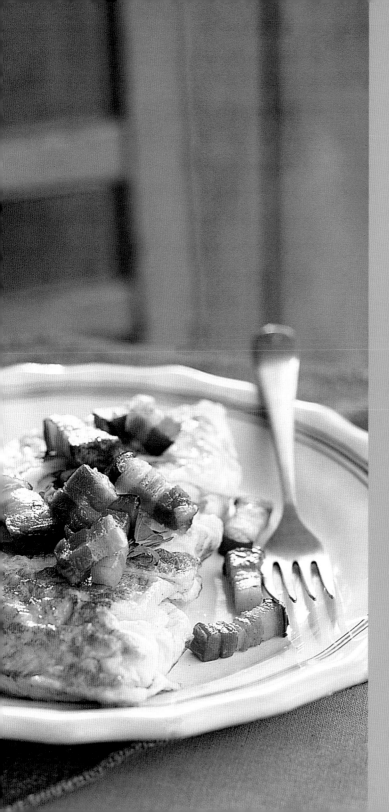

WHAT CAN I EAT?

The breakfast to the left is a good example of the protein-fat meal. It includes an omelette made with gruyère cheese, served with bacon and a cup of decaffeinated coffee. To create a completely different protein-fat breakfast, try combining any of the following elements.

For your protein element, choose from the following:
- eggs, any style
- fish, including smoked salmon
- meat, such as ham
- poultry, such as turkey or chicken

For your fat element, choose from the following:
- bacon
- cheese
- sausage

To drink, choose from the following:
- decaffeinated coffee
- pure Arabica coffee
- herbal or fruit tea

Lunch the Montignac way

Lunch is treated in much the same way as breakfast on the diet. That is, there are two flexible lunch options to choose from. Option 1 is a protein–fat meal, and this should be your staple lunch. It consists of protein-rich foods such as fish, meat, eggs, or poultry and carbohydrates with a GI no higher than 35. Option 2 is a high-fiber carbohydrate meal, composed of high-fiber, low to medium GI carbohydrates with a GI up to 50. This second type of meal should be limited to three to four times per week, and should never be eaten with saturated fats.

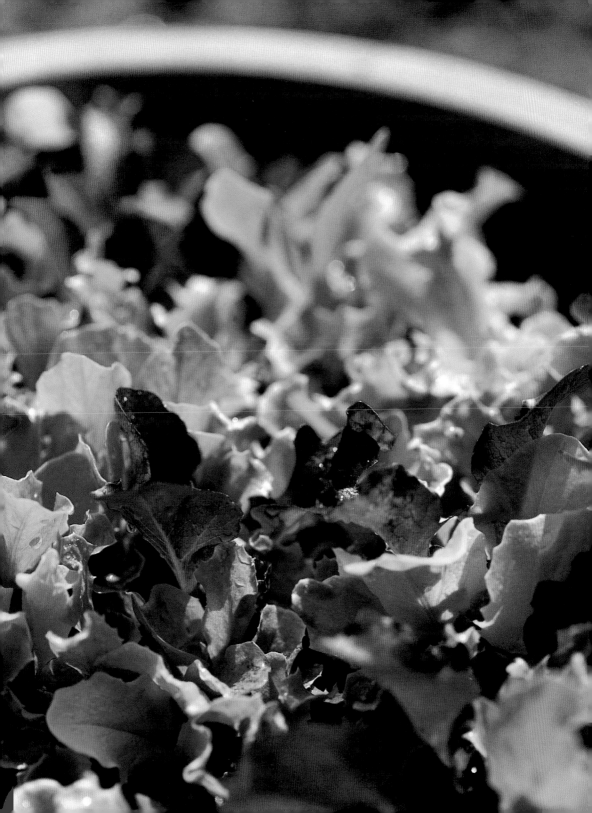

Option 1
protein-fat lunch

The Option 1 lunch is a staple meal on the Rapid Weight Loss Plan. It may consist of a soup, salad, and side dish made from carbohydrates with a GI of 35 or below, and protein, such as meat, poultry, eggs, or fish. These elements make it an ideal option for weight loss. Its success for slimming, however, hinges on eating only sub-35 GI carbohydrates.

SOUPS, STARTERS, AND SALADS

Start your meal with a soup made from vegetables with a very low GI value of 35 or below. Homemade soups such as gazpacho or mushroom soups are best, since commercially prepared soups may contain hidden sugars in the form of cornstarch and flour.

Other starters can be made up of a selection of vegetables with a sub-35 GI value. Feel free to use fats such as oil or butter when preparing this dish. For example, zucchini sautéed in olive oil would make an ideal starter for this type of meal. You can also have a side salad prepared with olive oil and cheese, such as leek and asparagus salad (*see pp166–67*). It's perfectly acceptable for these dishes to contain fat, so long as they do not include carbohydrates with a GI higher than 35.

MAIN COURSE

A dish containing a protein source, such as meat, fish, chicken, or eggs should be the main course in this type of meal. There are no restrictions on the type or amount of protein you choose, but they should always be prepared without bad carbohydrates, such as bread crumbs or flour. If you have high cholesterol, however, it is best to choose protein with a lower fat content, such as tofu, fish, skinless chicken, or lean pork. You can finish off your meal with a small glass of wine or beer and some cheese for dessert (*for more Rapid Weight Loss dessert options, see pp90–91*).

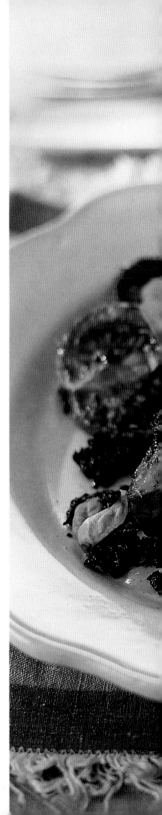

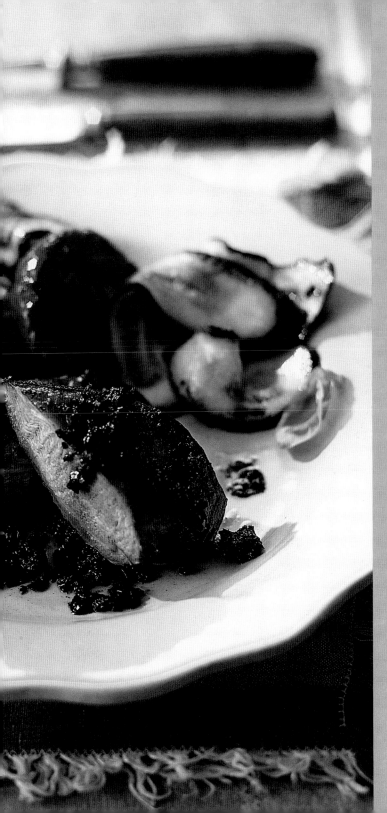

WHAT CAN I EAT?

The lunch to the left is a well-balanced protein-fat meal, consisting of roasted tomatoes and zucchini, which are low-GI carbohydrates, and lean grilled duck with a black olive tapenade, which fulfils the protein and fat requirements. Feel free to choose from the selection of foods below to create your ideal protein-fat meal. Remember, you can prepare these foods with fat, if you wish.

For your sub-35 GI carbohydrate element, choose from the following:
- low-GI vegetables, such as broccoli, peppers, and spinach
- low-GI legumes and grains, such as lentils, quinoa, or wild rice

For your protein element, choose from the following:
- meat
- fish
- poultry
- eggs
- soy products such as tofu

To drink, you can choose one of the following:
- still or sparkling water
- one 3.5-fl oz glass of wine or champagne
- one 3.5-fl oz glass of beer

Option 2
high-fiber carbohydrate lunch

This carbohydrate meal should contain minimal, if any, fat, and it should be eaten no more than 3 to 4 times per week. Like Option 1, it can include a soup, salad, and side dish made from very low-GI vegetables. For your main course, however, you can consume carbohydrates with a GI as high as 50.

SOUPS, STARTERS, AND SALADS

A broth-based soup made from vegetables with a sub-35 GI value is a great way to start this meal. If you use a canned soup, be vigilant: always scan the label to make sure it contains no hidden sugar or fat.

Your starter can include a selection of chopped or steamed vegetables with a sub-35 GI value. You should not add any saturated fats, such as butter, when preparing this dish. Steamed artichokes, for example, would make a filling and healthy side dish or starter for this meal. You can also have a salad prepared with a dressing made from nonfat yogurt, mustard, and lemon juice. Alternatively, you may drizzle a tiny bit of olive oil mixed with lemon juice or balsamic vinegar on your salad.

MAIN COURSE

Your main dish should be a high-fiber, sub-50 GI carbohydrate, so long as it is not bread (not even good, whole wheat bread). You might choose legumes, such as lentils, chickpeas, or haricot beans, brown or unrefined Basmati rice, or whole wheat spaghetti cooked *al dente*. Try some lentils cooked with onions and topped with fat-free natural yogurt or a bowl of whole wheat spaghetti cooked al dente, drizzled with a little olive oil. The fat you use should be minimal, and it should always be unsaturated. This means that this should be a meat-free meal. You may also have a small glass of wine or beer with your meal, followed by a low-fat dessert (*for more Rapid Weight Loss dessert options, see pp90–91*).

CAN I JUST EAT PASTA?

Unfortunately, no. This type of meal must include a range of very low-GI vegetables, in addition to pasta or any other medium-GI, high-fiber carbohydrate. Colorful vegetables, such as salad greens and tomatoes, provide your body with essential vitamins and minerals, and their very low GI values will help to bring down the total GI of your meal via the AGI principle (*see pp112–14*). So, enjoy your pasta or brown rice, and eat as much as you like, but whatever you do, don't forget to eat your vegetables!

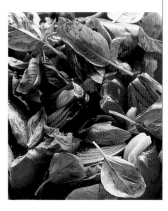

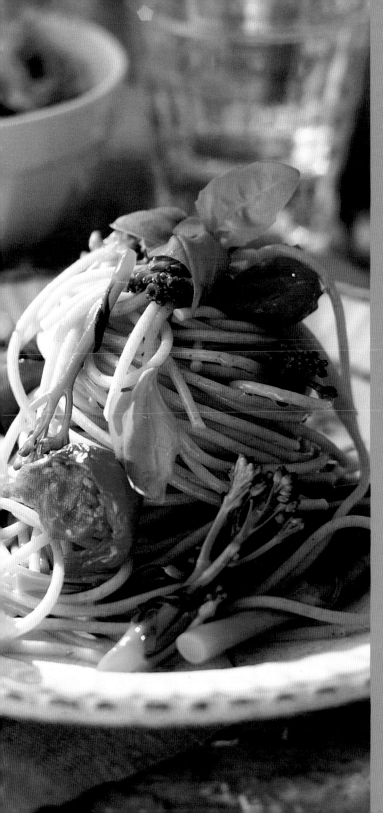

WHAT CAN I EAT?

The lunch to the left is a good example of a high-fiber carbohydrate meal. It includes whole wheat spaghetti (served cold) with herbs and vegetables, served with a side salad. Feel free to choose from the selection of foods below to create your ideal high-fiber carbohydrate meal. This meal should be prepared with very little fat; avoid saturated fat altogether.

For your sub-35 GI carbohydrate element, choose from the following:
- low-GI vegetables, such as broccoli, peppers, and spinach
- low-GI legumes and grains, such as lentils, quinoa, and wild rice

For your high-fiber carbohydrate element, choose from the following:
- whole wheat spaghetti (preferably served cold to reduce its GI value)
- legumes such as chickpeas, haricot beans, and kidney beans
- grains such as brown rice and unrefined Basmati rice

To drink, you can choose from one of the following:
- still or sparkling water
- one 3.5-fl oz glass of wine or champagne
- one 3.5-fl oz glass of beer

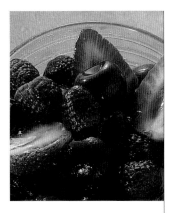

ON FRUIT

On the Rapid Weight Loss Plan, you can enjoy a range of desserts made from fruit, since most fruits have low GI values of 35 and below. Fresh fruit or fruit compote made from apples, pears, apricots, and peaches, for example, can be a delicious sweet treat after a meal. You can also enjoy fresh raspberries, cherries, and strawberries directly after your meal, since they also have low GI values. Another fruit-based option is to stir a bit of sugar-free jam into some low or nonfat yogurt or cream cheese. These low-fat desserts are ideal options following high-fiber carbohydrate meals.

On dessert

The main problem with classic desserts is that they are usually made with white flour, sugar, butter, or perhaps all three. But this does not mean that you have to forgo dessert completely when following the diet—you simply have to choose your desserts wisely.

CHOCOLATE AND OTHER SWEET TREATS

During the Rapid Weight Loss Plan, you may indulge in a wide variety of desserts. You must ensure, however, that the carbohydrates you use have a GI no higher than 35. Luckily, there are lots of healthy options open to you. For example, very few people know that dark chocolate (containing at least 70 percent cocoa) has a low GI of only 25. This means that you can enjoy a few squares of high-quality dark chocolate, or prepare desserts made from it, such as the decadent chocolate cake recipe listed at the back of this book (*see pp232–33*). It has a GI of 25, so you can enjoy it with a guilt-free conscience. So long as your sweet treat does not contain any food with a GI higher than 35, desserts are totally acceptable while following the Rapid Weight Loss Plan.

You can also eat desserts made with eggs, low-GI fruits (*see left*), and fructose, since these are all low-GI foods. If you creatively base your recipes around these simple ingredients, you can make a wide range of tasty desserts, such as Raspberry and chocolate mousse (*see p237*) and Chocolate vanilla pots (*see p236*).

If you take a lateral approach to creating Rapid Weight Loss desserts, there's an endless range of possibilities open to you. For example, you can devise your own flan recipe using my recipe for Cherry flan (from the *Montignac Provençal Cookbook*) as a template. Soak 1¾ pounds of stoned cherries in six tablespoons of rum. In a separate bowl, heat 7-fl ounces each of whipping cream and milk. Allow the milk and cream mixture to cool. In another bowl beat together six eggs, 2 ounces of fructose, and a drop of vanilla extract, and then add the milk and cream mixture to it, stirring constantly. Add the cherries and rum to this mixture and pour it into an 11-inch flan dish. Bake the flan at 265°F for 50 minutes and chill in the refrigerator before serving.

CHEESE FOR DESSERT

In France, cheese is accorded the honor of being eaten with a knife and fork—a practice that should be encouraged throughout the world. This is because almost all cheeses have a negligible GI value. In other words, cheese contains very little, if any, sugar, and it will not contribute to weight gain. After a protein-fat lunch or dinner, just about every cheese is allowed—provided you eat it on its own, without any carbohydrates.

In most restaurants, the menu offers a dessert or cheese option. When dining out on the Rapid Weight Loss Plan, you should limit yourself to the cheese option, since it's unlikely that any of the other desserts will be free from sugar and flour. Remember, though, you should always, always eat your cheese without bread or crackers. If you have high cholesterol, however, or if you have just eaten a high-fiber carbohydrate meal, you should only eat nonfat cheeses, such as nonfat cream cheese.

"In France, cheese is accorded the honor of being eaten with a knife and fork—a practice that should be encouraged throughout the world."

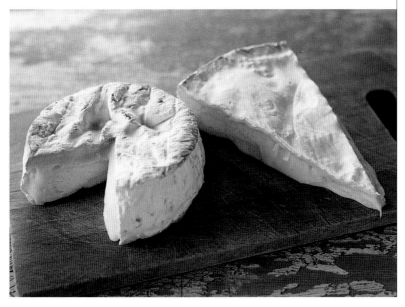

Left: *The French consider cheese, such as brie and camembert, a delicious treat for dessert.*

Dinner the Montignac way

Dinner on the diet is almost identical to lunch in that it gives you two meal options: a protein-fat meal or a high-fiber carbohydrate meal. These are the same meal guidelines you were given for lunch—the only difference is that your dinner should be lighter than your lunch. In other words, both options should have more low-GI vegetables and less fat or high-fiber carbohydrate than your lunch portion. One caveat: if you have had a high-fiber carbohydrate meal for lunch, then it is best to balance it out by having a protein-fat meal for dinner.

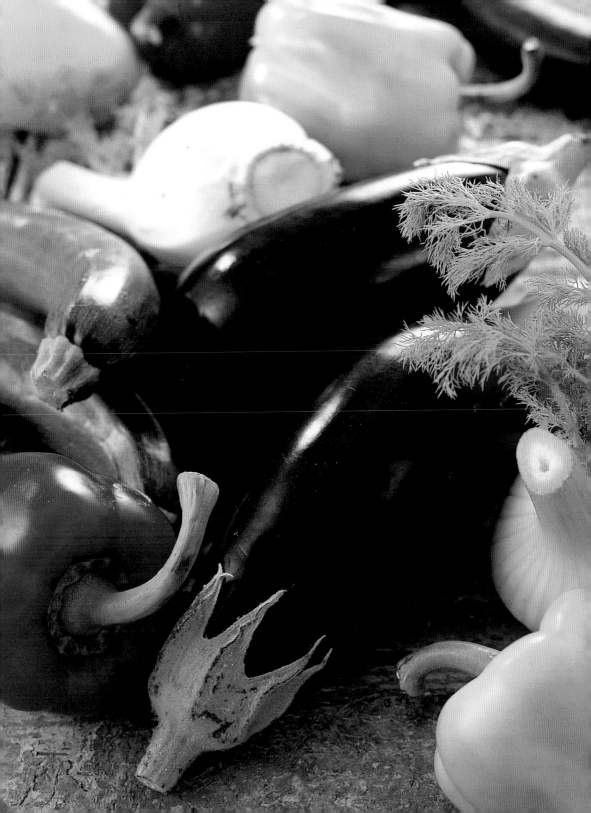

Option 1
protein-fat dinner

This dinner option is almost exactly the same as the protein-fat lunch (*see pp86–87*), but its proportions should shift slightly. That is, the protein-fat dinner should be prepared with less fat, and it should include more low-GI vegetables, than the protein-fat lunch. You should eat this type of dinner on most evenings, since it has a good balance of very low-GI carbohydrates, proteins, and fats. The golden rule, though, is to avoid carbohydrates with GI values higher than 35.

SOUPS, STARTERS, AND SALADS

These dishes should contain lots of very low-GI vegetables, and they should be lighter on fat than your lunch starters and salads. Your starter can be a soup consisting of very low-GI vegetables or a selection of grilled, sautéed, or roasted vegetables with a sub-35 GI value. You can also have a side salad containing vegetables with very low GI values. Remember, it's perfectly acceptable for these dishes to contain fat (albeit less than you used at lunchtime), as long as they do not include carbohydrates with a GI higher than 35.

MAIN COURSE

As with the protein-fat lunch, the main course for your protein-fat dinner should be composed of a protein food, such as meat, fish, eggs, or chicken (prepared without carbohydrates such as bread crumbs or flour). Your dinner portion should be smaller than your lunch, though. It is also best to avoid having fatty meats for dinner, if possible, particularly if you have already had fatty meat, such as steak, for lunch; choose fish or lean meats, such as skinless chicken or lean pork instead. Drink a small glass of wine or beer with your meal and have some cheese or dark chocolate for dessert (*for more Rapid Weight Loss dessert options, see pp90–91*).

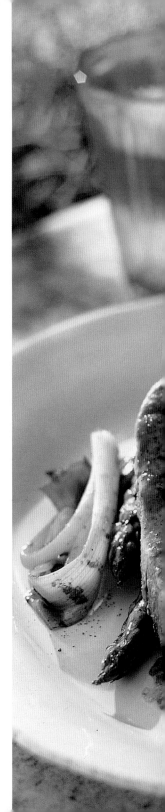

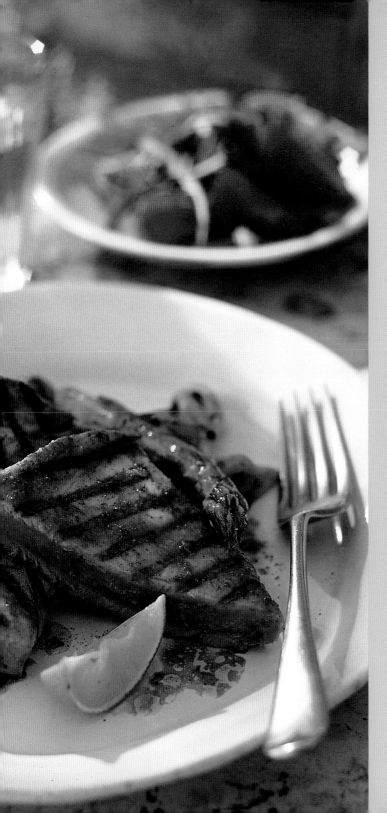

WHAT CAN I EAT?

The dinner to the left is a well-balanced, protein-fat meal, consisting of a tomato and arugula salad, grilled asparagus and spring onions (which are low-GI carbohydrates), and grilled tuna with Mediterranean marinade (*see pp200–01*), which fulfills the protein and fat requirements. Feel free to choose from the selection of foods below to create your ideal protein-fat dinner. Remember, you can prepare these foods with fat, if you wish.

For your sub-35 GI carbohydrate element, choose from the following:
- low-GI vegetables, such as broccoli, peppers, and spinach
- low-GI legumes and grains, such as lentils, quinoa, or wild rice

For your protein element, choose from the following:
- meat
- fish
- poultry
- eggs
- soy products, such as tofu

To drink, you can choose one of the following:
- still or sparkling water
- one 3.5-fl oz glass of wine or champagne
- one 3.5-fl oz glass of beer

Option 2
high-fiber carbohydrate dinner

This meal is very low in fat, and it should be eaten no more than 3 to 4 times per week. It allows you to eat carbohydrates with a GI as high as 50, as long as you eat them with little or no fat. To ensure a well-balanced diet, have this type of dinner only on days when you have had a protein-fat lunch.

SOUPS, STARTERS, AND SALADS

You can start this meal with a non-creamy broth or puréed soup made with vegetables with a sub-35 GI value. Alternatively, you can prepare a selection of raw or steamed vegetables with a sub-35 GI value, such as broccoli, peppers, and celery. Do not add any saturated fats, such as butter, when preparing these dishes. You can also have a salad prepared with a dressing made from nonfat yogurt, mustard, and lemon juice. Alternatively, you may drizzle a very little amount of olive oil mixed with lemon juice or balsamic vinegar on your salad. Use as little oil as possible—or better yet, skip it altogether.

MAIN COURSE

The main element of your meal should be a high-fiber carbohydrate with a GI of 50 or below. Your main dish can include lentils, brown rice, wild rice, chickpeas, or whole wheat spaghetti cooked *al dente*. A high-fiber carbohydrate main dish might be a mixed bean salad with peppers, tomatoes, and basil, drizzled with a little bit of olive oil.

   You should use very little, if any, fat when preparing this meal. If you do use a little oil, it should always be an unsaturated variety, such as olive oil. You may have a small 3.5-fl oz glass of wine, or a 3.5-fl oz glass of beer to drink with your meal. For dessert, avoid high-fat options, such as cheese, and instead choose something low in fat, such as nonfat cream cheese mixed with sugar-free jam.

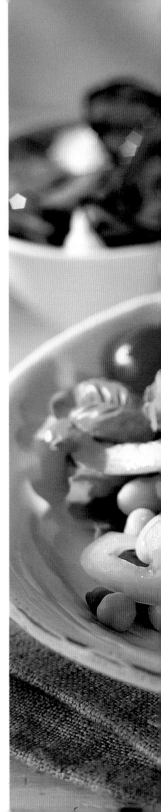

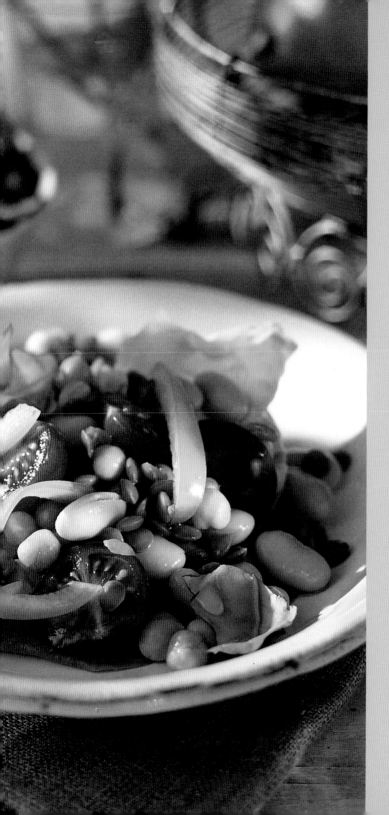

WHAT CAN I EAT?

The dinner to the left

is a well-balanced high-fiber carbohydrate meal. It includes a mixed bean salad with peppers, tomatoes, and basil, served with a side dish of grilled zucchini. Feel free to choose from the selection of foods below to create your ideal meal. This meal should be prepared with very little fat; avoid saturated fat altogether.

For your sub-35 GI

carbohydrate element, choose from the following:

- low-GI vegetables, such as broccoli, peppers, and spinach
- low-GI legumes and grains, such as lentils, quinoa, and wild rice

For your high-fiber

carbohydrate element, choose from the following:

- whole wheat spaghetti (preferably served cold to reduce its GI value)
- legumes such as chickpeas, haricot beans, and kidney beans
- grains such as brown rice and unrefined Basmati rice

To drink, you can choose one of the following:

- still or sparkling water
- one 3.5-fl oz glass of wine or champagne
- one 3.5-fl oz glass of beer

GRAB–AND–GO SNACKS

If you have not had time to prepare anything at home, you can always pop into a delicatessen and buy the foods you need over the counter. Italian delicatessens are particularly good for this option, since they stock a wide array of meats and cheeses, all of which contain little or no sugar. These snacks are high in saturated fat, so they cannot be eaten with bread—not even whole wheat bread.

For instance, you could buy:

• cooked or dried ham
I particularly recommend prosciutto, because it is cut very thinly, and any excess fat can be easily removed.

• turkey or chicken
It's best to choose skinless cuts of poultry whenever possible.

• dried sausage
Choose the leanest cut available and have it sliced for you in the shop, unless you happen to have a Swiss Army knife with you.

• hard-boiled eggs
If freshly prepared eggs aren't available, try them pickled.

• cheeses
All are suitable.

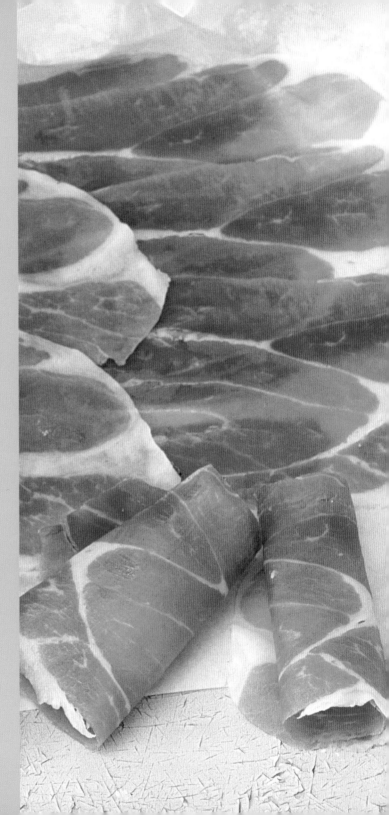

On snacks

If your afternoon meal has been sufficiently substantial, you should not feel the need to eat again before dinner. However, if you experience sharp hunger pangs, it is best to eat something. Whatever you do, never resort to eating high-GI carbohydrates, such as cookies, chips, bread, or popcorn. For weight loss, you must avoid carbohydrates with a GI above 35. The choices below are good snack options that will not undermine your weight loss plan.

PROTEIN IS ESSENTIAL

While it's important to choose very low-GI carbohydrates at snack time, the real key to keeping blood-sugar levels, and your appetite, under control is to include at least a little protein as well. As I said earlier in the book, protein, unlike carbohydrates, provides satiety, meaning it leaves you feeling fuller for longer than if you had eaten the same amount of carbohydrates (see pp24–25). It is for this reason that I recommend choosing protein-based snack foods, such as meat or cheese, in addition to your sub-35, low-GI carbohydrates.

Always be prepared!

Planning balanced snacks in advance can prevent you from making unhealthy snack choices. An ideal Rapid Weight Loss snack could include chopped raw vegetables, such as carrots, celery, tomatoes, and peppers, as well as slices of lean meats, and some cheese, such as cheddar or gruyère. All of these foods can be eaten freely, since they have very low GI values.

Prepare this snack ahead of time, and carry it with you in a sealed plastic container. This way, you can head off dietary disaster and avoid grabbing some cookies and a cola in hunger-fueled, hypoglycemic desperation. If you're caught unprepared, you can always stop by a delicatessen and buy something there (see panel, left).

MEAT-FREE SNACKS

For a fast and easy option, you could have a snack consisting entirely of fresh or dried fruits with a GI of 35 or below. Eat as much as you like. The problem, however, with fruit is that it is quickly digested and you may soon feel hungry again. That is why for a grab-and-go snack I recommend eating something more substantial, which contains protein, since the body digests protein more slowly than carbohydrates. Try nuts such as almonds, hazelnuts, or walnuts. A low-fat liquid yogurt is another good snack option that contains protein.

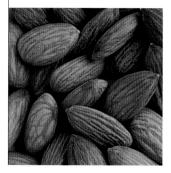

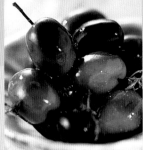

rapid weight loss
socializing

don't put a damper on party proceedings (or well-meaning friends who may cajole you into drinking with them). Don't tell anyone that you're abstaining from cocktails.

raise your glass to your lips as often as you would normally drink, but instead of drinking the alcohol, simply moisten your lips.

buy the first round of drinks, when out with your friends. Buy yourself a sparkling water with lime or a glass of tomato juice. As far as your friends know, you're drinking a vodka tonic or a Bloody Mary!

_____ **choose red or white wine** or champagne over spirits for your apéritif, if you must drink. Wine and champagne contain less alcohol than spirits, and therefore they present less risk of jeopardizing your weight loss regime.

_____ **accept a glass of good champagne** before your meal, should you be unable to do otherwise. Eat a few tidbits first, though, provided they do not contain any bad carbohydrates.

_____ **break open your roll** and then leave it uneaten on the side of your plate when at dinner parties. No one will notice!

_____ **indulge in cheese,** olives, delicatessen meats, smoked fish, or smoked eel when faced with the canapés tray. Eat something, and then enjoy your glass of champagne or wine, guilt-free.

Rapid Weight Loss menu plan

If you need some inspiration for planning your Rapid Weight Loss meals and snacks, you can refer to the following sample seven-day menu plan for ideas.

This menu maps out a balanced variety of meals for each day. It includes three high-fiber carbohydrate meals, but you can have four, if you wish.

MEAL	DAY 1	DAY 2	DAY 3
Breakfast with herbal *or* fruit tea *or* decaffeinated coffee	• sugarfree oat clusters with skim milk and strawberries	• whole wheat toast with sugarfree jam • low-fat natural yogurt with raspberries	• rice cakes topped with nonfat cheese and sliced apples
Lunch with one 3.5-fl oz glass dry wine *or* one 3.5-fl oz glass beer	• Greek salad (salad greens, feta cheese, tomatoes, onions, and olive oil) • omelette made with Emmental cheese • a few squares of dark chocolate	• vegetable soup, e.g. broccoli soup • grilled zucchini • Tricolor rice with balsamic onions (*see p193*); mashed cauliflower • apples with cinnamon	• Cherry tomato soup with basil (*see pp160–61*) • chef salad (salad greens, cheese, ham, boiled egg, tomatoes, and olive oil) • a few squares of dark chocolate
Snack (optional)	• sugar-free yogurt drink	• egg salad and crudités	• almonds and hazelnuts
Dinner with one 3.5-fl oz glass dry wine *or* one 3.5-fl oz glass beer	• vegetable soup, e.g. puréed cucumber soup • green salad • grilled cod; sautéed broccoli • Peach mousse (*see pp234–35*)	• Soupe au vin blanc (*see p162*) • Pork with herbed mustard (*see pp228–29*); steamed artichokes • sliced peaches with fromage frais	• vegetable soup, e.g. puréed zucchini soup • Wild mushroom custards (*see pp184–85*); arugula salad • chopped apples with cream cheese

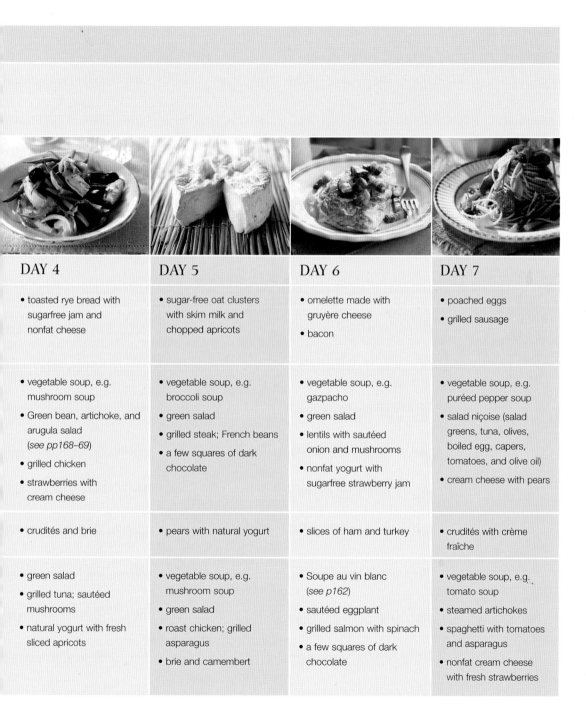

DAY 4

- toasted rye bread with sugarfree jam and nonfat cheese

- vegetable soup, e.g. mushroom soup
- Green bean, artichoke, and arugula salad (see pp168–69)
- grilled chicken
- strawberries with cream cheese

- crudités and brie

- green salad
- grilled tuna; sautéed mushrooms
- natural yogurt with fresh sliced apricots

DAY 5

- sugar-free oat clusters with skim milk and chopped apricots

- vegetable soup, e.g. broccoli soup
- green salad
- grilled steak; French beans
- a few squares of dark chocolate

- pears with natural yogurt

- vegetable soup, e.g. mushroom soup
- green salad
- roast chicken; grilled asparagus
- brie and camembert

DAY 6

- omelette made with gruyère cheese
- bacon

- vegetable soup, e.g. gazpacho
- green salad
- lentils with sautéed onion and mushrooms
- nonfat yogurt with sugarfree strawberry jam

- slices of ham and turkey

- Soupe au vin blanc (see p162)
- sautéed eggplant
- grilled salmon with spinach
- a few squares of dark chocolate

DAY 7

- poached eggs
- grilled sausage

- vegetable soup, e.g. puréed pepper soup
- salad niçoise (salad greens, tuna, olives, boiled egg, capers, tomatoes, and olive oil)
- cream cheese with pears

- crudités with crème fraîche

- vegetable soup, e.g. tomato soup
- steamed artichokes
- spaghetti with tomatoes and asparagus
- nonfat cream cheese with fresh strawberries

Selection of good carbohydrates

Since carbohydrates are the only foods that contain sugar, GI values apply only to these foods. Fats and proteins contain very little sugar and their impact on blood sugar levels is negligible (*see pp22–31*). The following is a small selection of good carbohydrate choices for the Rapid Weight Loss Plan.

Food	GI	Food	GI
Avocados	10	Peppers (green)	15
Almonds	15	Peppers (red)	15
Asparagus	15	Peppers (yellow)	15
Artichokes	15	Pumpkin seeds	15
Brazil nuts	15	Spinach	15
Broccoli	15	Sunflower seeds	15
Brussels sprouts	15	Walnuts	15
Cabbage (all kinds)	15	Zucchini	15
Cauliflower	15	Eggplant	20
Celery root	15	Fructose	20
Celery	15	Lemons	20
Cucumber	15	Limes	20
Fennel	15	Chinese vermicelli (soybean variety)	22
Hazelnuts	15	Beans, flageolet	25
Herbs	15	Blackberries	25
Leeks	15	Cherries	25
Lettuce (all kinds)	15	Dark chocolate (70 percent cocoa)	25
Mushrooms	15	Lentils (green)	25
Olives (all kinds)	15	Raspberries	25
Onions (all kinds)	15	Soybeans (cooked)	25
Peanuts	15	Split peas (yellow, cooked for 20 minutes)	25
Pecans	15	Strawberries	25

Apples (fresh)	30		Peas (dried, cooked)	35
Apricots (fresh)	30		Peas (fresh, cooked)	35
Beans, fresh green or string beans	30		Plums	35
Carrots (raw)	30		Prunes	35
Chickpeas (garbanzo beans), cooked	30		Quinoa	35
Fruit jam (sugarfree)	30		Satsumas	35
Garlic	30		Wild rice	35
Grapefuit	30		Figs (dried)	40
Lentils (brown)	30			
Lentils (red)	30		**For the carbohydrate-protein breakfast, only:**	
Lentils (yellow)	30		Black bread (German)	40
Milk (1% low-fat or skim)	30		Bread made from unrefined flour	40
Mung beans (soaked and cooked for 20 minutes)	30		Rye bread	45
Nectarines	30		Whole wheat bread with bran	45
Peaches	30			
Pears	30		**For high-fiber carbohydrate meals, only:**	
Tomatoes	30		Rice (unrefined Basmati)	50
Apples (dried)	35		Rice (brown)	50
Apricots (dried)	35		Sweet potatoes	50
Beans, broad (peeled and cooked)	35		Spaghetti, durum wheat (cooked *al dente*)	40
Beans, haricot	35		Spaghetti, whole wheat (cooked *al dente*)	40
Figs (fresh)	35			
Kidney beans	35			
Natural yogurt	35			
Oranges	35			

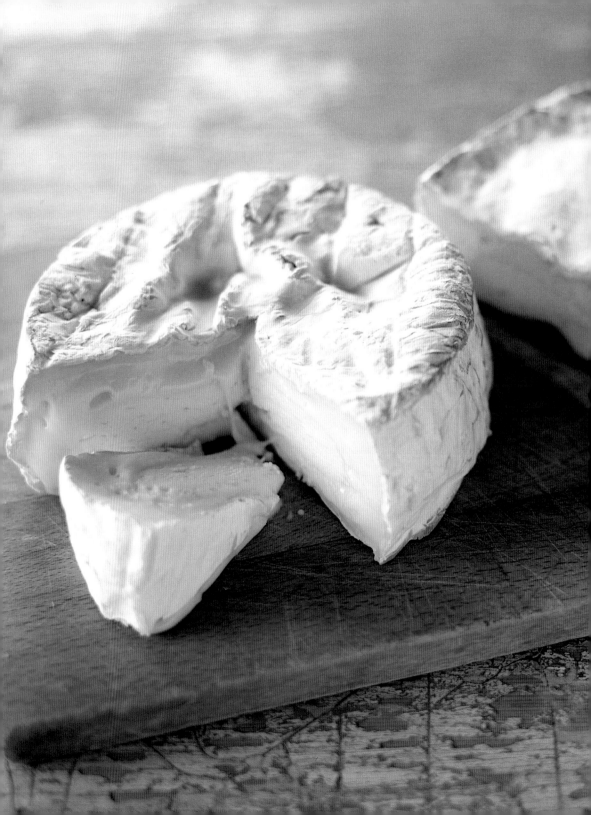

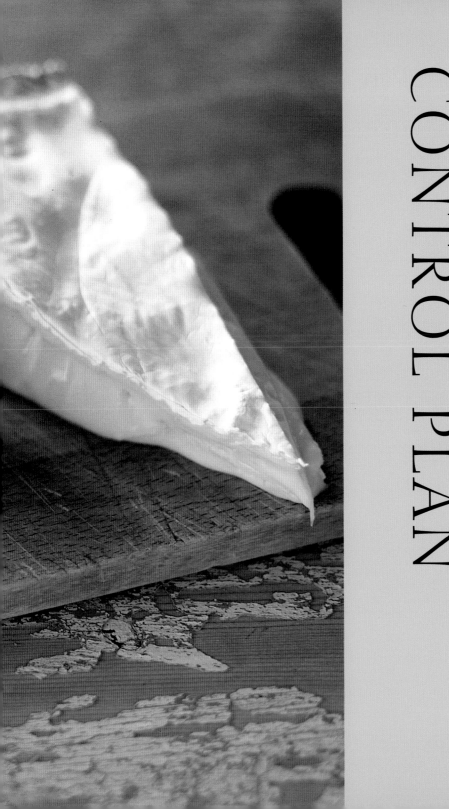

WEIGHT
CONTROL PLAN

In a nutshell

This next section introduces you to some of the new rules you will be following on the Weight Control Plan. The first thing you are likely to notice is that there are not many rules at all. That is because the defining characteristic of this plan is flexibility. In fact, it is more a guide to good, healthy living, inspired by the French way of life. The longer you stay on the Weight Control Plan, the easier choosing the right foods and maintaining your weight will become.

THE OBJECTIVES

The main purpose of the Weight Control Plan is weight maintenance. That said, the Weight Control Plan can be used in two different ways: firstly, it can be used after the Rapid Weight Loss Plan to maintain your new weight and healthy pancreas. Secondly, if weight loss is not your main objective, you can skip the Rapid Weight Loss Plan altogether, and jump straight into the Weight Control Plan to maintain your current weight and the health of your pancreas.

Weight maintenance

On the Weight Control Plan, you may eat carbohydrates with a GI of up to 50 without gaining weight. Following this rule, as well as the other guidelines for this plan, will allow you to maintain your weight. If you have just lost weight on the Rapid Weight Loss Plan, you should approach the Weight Control Plan not as a separate eating plan, but instead as a more moderate and flexible extension of the Rapid Weight Loss Plan. It is important for you to stick to most of the rules from the Rapid Weight Loss Plan and gradually incorporate the new elements from the Weight Control Plan over a period of a few weeks (*see pp48–49*). If you are simply interested in maintaining your current weight, and are starting the diet with the Weight Control Plan, by all means implement all of the rules at once.

"The longer you stay on the Weight Control Plan, the easier choosing the right foods and maintaining your weight will become."

The healthy pancreas

Now that you have a healthy pancreas, it is essential that you maintain it properly. If you slip into poor eating habits of eating bad, high-GI carbohydrates, your pancreas will become unwell. This will result in your entering a state of hyperinsulinism, and its accompanying sluggishness and weight gain.

Remember, being overweight is not caused by eating too much, but by eating the wrong foods. This, in turn, causes the body to produce too much insulin and store excess glucose as fat. If you follow the Weight Control guidelines, however, your pancreas should remain in good condition. In fact, the longer you follow the diet, the better your pancreas will function, the easier it will be to maintain your weight, and the more relaxed you can be with your food choices.

Eat sub-50 GI for weight maintenance

The Weight Control Plan encourages you to eat a wide variety of high-quality, delicious foods, and there are fewer rules and restrictions than on the Rapid Weight Loss Plan. If you want to maintain your weight and the health of your pancreas, you must always choose foods with a GI of 50 or below. If you do eat a carbohydrate with a GI higher than this, minimize the damage by implementing the AGI principle and eating a very low-GI carbohydrate first (*see pp112–14*). The diagram below shows how your weight is affected by the GI of the foods you eat.

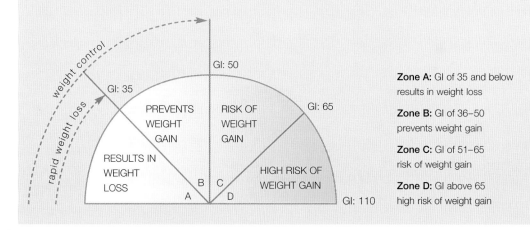

Zone A: GI of 35 and below results in weight loss

Zone B: GI of 36–50 prevents weight gain

Zone C: GI of 51–65 risk of weight gain

Zone D: GI above 65 high risk of weight gain

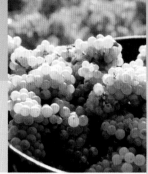

weight control

the rules

1   **maintain your weight** with this plan. It is actually a flexible extension of the Rapid Weight Loss Plan. If you do not wish to lose weight, however, you can skip the Rapid Weight Loss Plan, and jump straight into the Weight Control Plan to maintain your weight and the health of your pancreas.

2   **keep both breakfast options:** the protein-carbohydrate breakfast and the protein-fat breakfast. The protein-carbohydrate breakfast is the healthier option and you should have it on most mornings.

3   **you may eat flexible main meals.** In other words, there are no more "meal options" for lunch or dinner. There is really one golden rule to bear in mind: always choose carbohydrates with a GI of 50 or below. If you want to include a carbohydrate with a GI higher than this, you must count it as a discrepancy (*see opposite and pp116–17*) or use the AGI principle (*see opposite and pp112–14*).

4 **eat whole grain bread** as part of the carbohydrate-protein breakfast and as a snack. However, because all bread, even good, whole grain bread, is very high in starch, these are the only times bread can be eaten on the Weight Control Plan.

5 **use the AGI principle,** or the average glycemic index, if you want to eat a carbohydrate with a GI higher than 50 (*see pp112–14*). It will reduce the effects of the high-GI food on your blood-sugar levels.

6 **you can have two high–GI treats,** or discrepancies, per month without running the risk of gaining weight (*see pp116–17*). This involves planning a chosen treat in advance, and minimizing the effects through a specially tailored plan of action.

7 **have two small glasses of wine** or one 12-fl oz bottle of beer with your main meals each day, if you wish. You may have the occasional apéritif or after-dinner drink, in moderation (*see pp128–29*). Whatever you do, however, you must never drink alcohol on an empty stomach.

What is the AGI?

Eating good food is one of the supreme experiences of our existence, and cooking is a true art, in the same league as music or painting. This is why it would be a pity to deprive oneself forever of foods that, despite the fact that they may have a relatively high GI value, nonetheless have an important gastronomic dimension. By implementing the AGI (average glycemic index) principle, you will be able to eat some of these delicacies without gaining weight.

WHAT IS THE AGI PRINCIPLE?

The AGI is one of the most important aspects of the Weight Control Plan. It is exactly what its name suggests: the average GI of all the carbohydrates eaten during the course of a meal. So, it is not the GI value of any one particular carbohydrate you eat during a meal that matters most, but the combined effect that several carbohydrate foods have on one another. So, if you happen to eat a high-GI carbohydrate during the course of a meal, the outcome will not necessarily be a catastrophe for your blood-sugar levels and your weight.

How does the AGI principle work?

The AGI is, in essence, your body's system of checks and balances, and it will allow you to eat certain high-GI foods, so long as they are accompanied (or preferably preceded by) some very low-GI, high-fiber carbohydrates. This means that if you eat a carbohydrate with a GI that is slightly higher than recommended (above 50 on the Weight Control Plan), its effect on your pancreas will be reduced by eating another carbohydrate that has a very low GI value.

So, for example, a dish of potatoes will cause the glucose level in your blood to rise appreciably, whereas low-GI vegetables rich in fiber will cause glucose levels to rise only slightly. Eat the two together and the

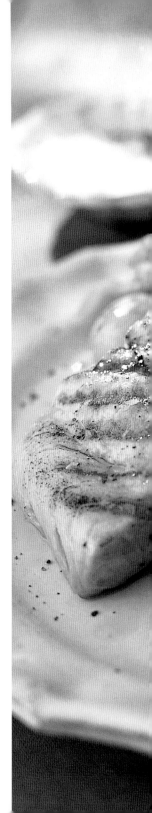

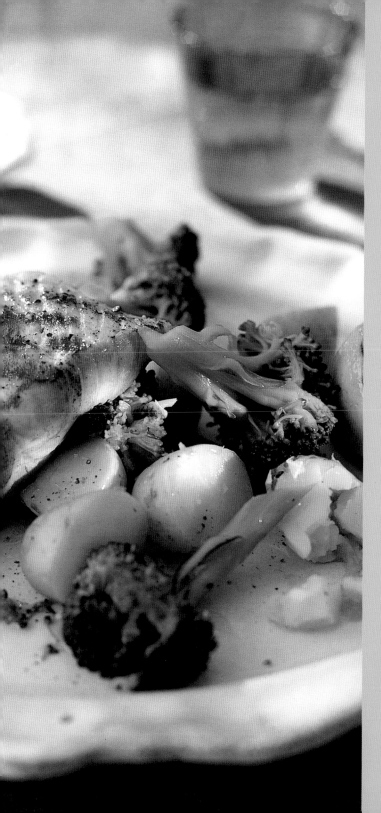

THE AGI IN ACTION

This meal (see left) is a good illustration of the AGI principle. The formula below is not an exact science. It should only be used to get an approximation of the AGI, and not an exact figure. The dinner includes boiled potatoes (a very high-GI food), steamed broccoli (a very low-GI food), and grilled salmon. The broccoli will bring down the AGI of the potatoes, so long as you eat your carbohydrates in this order:

• the broccoli should be eaten first, since it has a low GI of 15. Its low GI will bring down the high GI of the potatoes.

• the potatoes should be eaten next. They have been boiled in their skins and have a high GI of 65.
Add this GI value to that of the broccoli, and you get 80. To get an average glycemic index, or AGI, divide by two.

• the AGI of the two foods, when eaten together, is about 40, which is a perfectly acceptable AGI on the Weight Control Plan.

• it is worth noting that the AGI should only be obtained through eating normal quantities of low-GI foods to compensate for high-GI foods, not huge amounts.

glucose level in your blood will increase to a level somewhere between the two extremes, depending on how much of the potato and how many of the low-GI, high-fiber vegetables you have eaten.

The limits of the AGI

This is not a cut-and-dried formula, and it should be viewed as a guideline only for how to eat carbohydrates with a GI higher than 50 on the Weight Control Plan. To offset the potential damage of a high-GI food, you must always aim to implement the AGI principle by eating a very low-GI carbohydrate *before* you eat your high-GI carbohydrate. The order in which you eat your carbohydrates is key. If you eat your high-GI carbohydrate first, your blood sugar levels will remain high.

The AGI principle is a general guideline, and moderation is the key to using it to maintaining your weight. Too many carbohydrates, regardless of their GI values, will be transformed into body fat. If you eat a huge portion of potatoes, you should not eat an enormous portion of broccoli to "undo" the damage. You must consider not just the AGI, but also the concentration of carbohydrates contained in your meal.

The concentration of carbohydrates

The GI of a carbohydrate is important, but it needs to be seen in relation to the concentration of carbohydrate—that is, the number of ounces of carbohydrates that a food contains. The chart to the right reveals a few pleasant surprises. For instance, a cooked carrot has a high GI value of 85, but it has a low carbohydrate content of 6 grams per 3.5 ounce (100 gram) serving. French fried potatoes, however, have a high concentration of carbohydrate of 33 grams per serving.

So, a small portion of cooked carrots will have a minimal effect on your blood-sugar levels. You would have to eat nearly 21 ounces of cooked carrots to achieve the same blood-sugar spike as 3.5 ounces of potatoes. Other high-GI, low-carbohydrate foods include melon (6g), turnips (3g), and watermelon (7g). On this plan, you do not have to be as vigilant about these foods. Provided you do not eat them too often and in too great a quantity, they will not cause you to gain weight.

"Eating good food is one of the supreme experiences of our existence, and cooking is a true art, in the same league as music or painting."

Concentration of carbohydrates

The concentration of carbohydrate is the number of grams of carbohydrate contained in a 3.5 ounce (100 gram) serving of food. Foods with a high GI, but a low carbohydrate concentration (10g or less per serving), are fine to eat in moderation, and are marked by an asterisk below.

Food	Carbohydrate concentration	GI	Food	Carbohydrate concentration	GI
Apricots (dried)	63g	35	Lentils (green)	17g	25
Apricots (fresh)	10g	30	Melon*	6g	60
Bananas	20g	60	Milk (1% low-fat)	5g	30
Beans, fresh green or string beans	3g	30	Natural (unflavored) yogurt	5g	35
Beans, haricot	17g	35	Peanuts	9g	15
Beets*	10g	65	Peas, dried	7g	35
Carrots (cooked)*	6g	85	Potato (fried or french fried)	33g	95
Carrots (raw)	6g	30	Pumpkin*	7g	75
Chickpeas (garbanzo beans)	22g	30	Quinoa	35g	18
Chinese vermicelli, soybean variety	15g	22	Raisins (dark or golden)	66g	65
Cornflakes	85g	85	Rice (unrefined Basmati)	23g	50
Dark chocolate (70 percent cocoa)	32g	25	Rice (brown)	23g	50
Flour	53g	70	Rice cakes	24g	85
Fructose	100g	20	Rice (pre-cooked, long grain)	24g	70
Grapes (all kinds)	16g	45	Soybeans (cooked)	15g	25
Honey	80g	85	Sweet potato	20g	50
Jam (made with sugar)	70g	65	Sugar (saccharose)	100g	70
Jam (sugarfree)	37g	30	Sultanas	66g	65
Kidney beans	11g	35	Spaghetti, durum wheat (al dente)	25g	40
Kiwi	12g	50	Turnips*	3g	70
Lentils (brown; red; yellow)	17g	30	Watermelon*	7g	75

Q&A

What are discrepancies?

This aspect of the diet is closely tied to the AGI principle (*see pp112–14*). It is also one of the diet's most subtle and complicated concepts to put into practice. Make sure you have a good understanding of the AGI before incorporating any discrepancies into your diet.

Q What exactly is a discrepancy?

A discrepancy is a planned deviation from the diet. It allows you to occasionally eat foods with a GI much higher than 50. A discrepancy is not a binge or a failure of will because it is planned and deliberate. It is unique to this plan because your pancreas should be well enough to cope with the occasional high–GI food.

Q Is there anything I can't have?

No. Any relatively high–GI food may be considered a discrepancy, providing it fulfils two conditions: firstly, the food must be a genuine exception to the way you normally eat. Secondly, you should take into account the food's GI and its concentration of carbohydrates, and whenever possible, choose the "least bad" option.

Q How often can I include discrepancies?

I am loath to discuss discrepancies because people can misuse the concept and gain weight. Remember, this is your chance to enjoy your favorite foods, without guilt, on very special occasions. Therefore, it is essential that you do not abuse your discrepancy privilege, and that you limit them to no more than twice a month.

Q Is there a golden rule on discrepancies?

Yes. If you are planning to have a discrepancy, always finish your meal with one and never start with one. If you begin your meal with low-GI foods, followed by a high-GI food, the average GI will remain relatively low, stimulating a minimal insulin response. A high-GI food eaten at the beginning of the meal will cause blood-sugar levels to remain high, even if you then eat a low-GI food. So, have dessert after dinner, but never have bread before your meal.

Q How do I incorporate my discrepancies?

The trick is to deliberately plan to have your treat, and exercise caution in your other food choices. For example, if you know you want a regular dessert (e.g. a slice of pie) after dinner, that is your planned discrepancy. Simply make certain that the rest of your meal contains very low-GI carbohydrates (and lean protein, for added satiety). Eat your low-GI, healthy carbohydrates first. Then, you should enjoy your dessert, guilt-free, and savor every mouthful. The presence of high-fiber, low-GI carbohydrates will offset the damage done by lowering the AGI of your meal.

Q Are there any caveats?

Ideally, your discrepancies should consist of foods with a low concentration of carbohydrates, such as watermelon, since their impact on blood sugar levels is easier to balance out. But once you start distinguishing between big and small discrepancies, you run the risk of focusing your undivided attention on the big ones, while overlooking the small ones. Never lose sight of the fact that small discrepancies are still deviations, and they should not become a regular feature in your diet or you will gain weight.

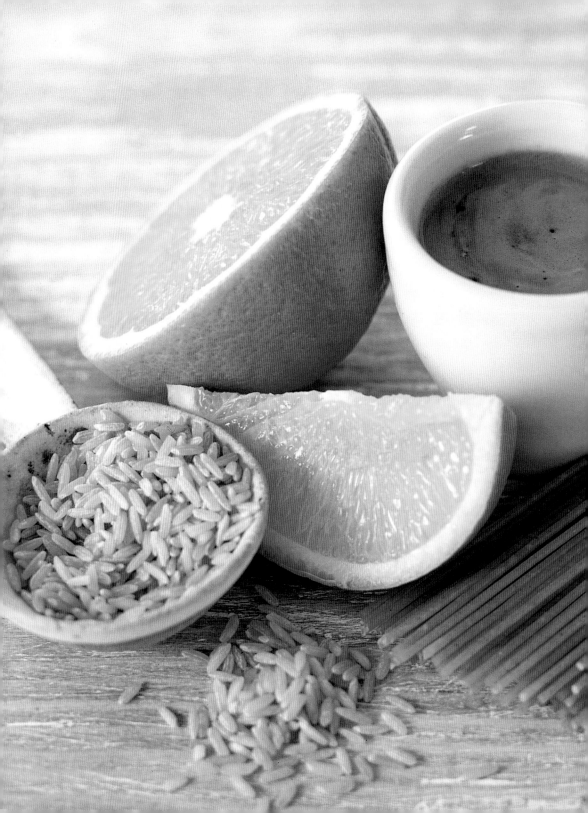

Choose foods wisely

The Weight Control Plan is a more relaxed extension of the Rapid Weight Loss Plan (*see pp44–105*), but there are still some foods that should be treated with caution. This section will show you how to choose the right foods to maintain your weight.

- starches

- bread

- pasta

- fruit

- drinks

On starches

Even on the Weight Control Plan, I remain staunchly opposed to certain starches, such as white potatoes, sticky white rice, and corn. These foods have high GI values, and eating them regularly will invariably lead to weight gain. However, not all starches are bad for you, and on this plan you can enjoy all of the good starches without rules or restrictions.

POTATOES

Sweet potatoes are rich in fiber, which gives them a medium GI of 50. This GI value makes sweet potatoes an acceptable food to eat freely on the Weight Control Plan. Always eat them with the skin on to retain their fiber content and to ensure that their GI does not rise above 50.

A white potato, on the other hand, can have a GI value as high as 95, since it contains very little in the way of fiber. Given their high GI, it almost goes without saying that white potatoes are terrible for your weight, and should be avoided at all costs. If you must have potatoes, though, do so rarely, and always employ the AGI principle by eating some very low-GI, high-fiber vegetables first.

RICE AND OTHER GRAINS

Unrefined Basmati rice, brown rice, and wild rice are rich in fiber and they all have GI values of 50 and below. This means that you may eat any of these foods whenever you wish on the Weight Control Plan. Wild rice, which is actually an oat and not a rice, is especially good since it has a very low GI of 35. Quinoa is another recommended low-GI grain option, since it also has a GI of 35.

Refined regular sticky white rice, however, is almost completely devoid of fiber. Its high-starch, low-fiber content gives it a very high GI of at least 70, which is roughly the same GI as sugar itself. So, this kind of white rice is banned, even on the Weight Control Plan. If you do eat white rice, do so on rare occasions, and always consider it a discrepancy.

PASTA

The Weight Control Plan permits you to eat pasta whenever you like, and not just as a part of certain specified meals. You can also eat white pasta, so long as it is made from durum wheat. If you are unsure if a pasta is made from durum wheat, then stick with whole wheat pasta, which is a safe, relatively low-GI option. The best pastas are pastified varieties, such as spaghetti and linguini (*see pp64–65*). Even better is Chinese vermicelli, made from soy flour. It has a very low GI of 22, which is the lowest GI of all pastas. Always cook your pasta so that it is *al dente*.

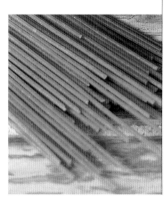

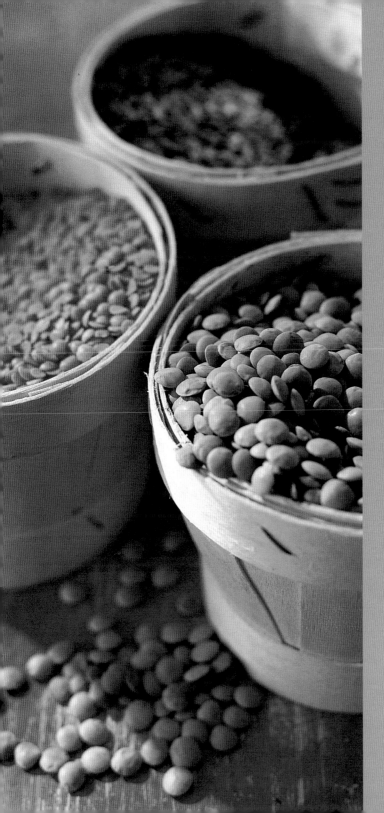

LEGUMES

All types of lentils and other legumes, such as chickpeas, haricot beans, French beans, and split peas, can be eaten freely throughout both plans of the Diet since they have very low GI values. Green, red, yellow, and brown lentils are particularly good choices, since their GI values are very low, ranging from 25 to 30. Kidney beans have a slightly higher GI value of 35, but they, too, can be eaten freely without fear of weight gain. All of these legumes are relatively low-GI foods that are high in fiber and can be eaten whenever you wish.

Can I eat bread?

Be careful with bread, even on the Weight Control Plan. Some types of breads are very high in starch (with a carbohydrate concentration of 53 grams per 3.5 ounce/100 gram serving) and sugar, and if you abuse them, you run the risk of destabilizing your pancreas and gaining weight. If you have lost weight on the Rapid Weight Loss Plan, this Q&A section will give you the information you need to help you avoid regaining the weight you have lost.

Q Is bread still fattening on this plan?

The answer is a qualified yes. Certain types of bread, such as white bread, baguettes, rolls, and croissants, will always wreak havoc on your waistline. Although your pancreas should be functioning properly, even a healthy pancreas cannot handle the burden of sugar and starch present in these high-GI breads. If you indulge in these foods no more than twice a month, as planned discrepancies (*see pp116-17*), then you should not experience any problems. Exceeding this limit, however, will destabilize your pancreas so that it secretes too much insulin, which will lead to weight gain.

Q Can I still eat bread for breakfast?

Yes. For the carbohydrate-protein breakfast, you should continue to eat only unrefined whole grain or rye bread. After about three months on the Weight Control Plan, you may spread your bread with a little light margarine, if you wish. When eating your protein-fat breakfast option, however, you should avoid eating any bread—even if it happens to be good whole grain bread!

Q What kind of bread can I eat?

The good breads are rye or whole grain varieties, preferably made from unrefined, organic flour. However, white bread will always be banned from the diet, even on the Weight Control Plan. No matter how healthy your pancreas may be, regularly including white bread in your diet will always lead to weight gain and metabolic imbalance. During breakfast, lunch, or dinner, at home, at the cafeteria, or in a good restaurant, you should always obey the golden rule: no white bread!

Q When else can I eat bread?

On the Weight Control Plan, you can eat unrefined whole grain or rye bread not just for breakfast, but as a snack, too. These are the only times that bread is permitted. The snack is something I call the Sandwich à la Montignac (*see pp144–45*). The bread should be whole grain or rye and it should be toasted, since toasting bread may reduce its GI value. Fill the sandwich with very low-GI vegetables, lean meats, and nonfat cheeses. Remember, this is a snack, not a side dish and it should be eaten only on an empty stomach.

Q Can I never eat another croissant?

If you love croissants or white bread, then make these foods one of your two discrepancies a month and it is unlikely that you will gain weight. On occasion, I find it impossible to resist delicious (but very high-GI) croissants oozing with butter. In such instances, at the end of the meal, I automatically take into account how my dietary balance has been upset. In other words, I will usually make a mental note of what I had for breakfast, and eat prudently and sensibly for the rest of the day.

On fruit

Whether you are on the Weight Control Plan or Rapid Weight Loss Plan, sugar is considered poison on the diet. Although fruit is full of vitamins and fiber, it also contains some sugar. It is therefore essential to monitor the GI of every piece of fruit you eat. Fortunately, most fruits have low GI values, and are therefore not only acceptable on the Weight Control Plan, but are recommended.

FRESH AND DRIED FRUIT

The rules for eating fruit on the Rapid Weight Loss Plan (*see pp66–67*) also apply here. That is, you can eat fresh fruit, but be wary of its GI value. On the Rapid Weight Loss Plan, you were only allowed those fresh fruits with a GI value of 35 and below. On the Weight Control Plan, you may eat fruits with a GI as high as 50, but no higher than that. Luckily, most fresh fruits, such as apples, apricots, cherries, figs, and pears, have GI values that fall far below this limit. You can also enjoy kiwi and grapes, which have GI values of 50 and 45, respectively. The list of high-GI fresh fruits is fortunately short, and it includes fruits such as melon and watermelon. Although these fruits have high GI values, because their concentration of carbohydrates (*see pp114–15*) is low, you may eat these foods in moderation on the Weight Control Plan.

Uncooked dried fruits have a medium GI but contain a lot of good fiber. This means that they are ideal if you do a lot of vigorous exercise, such as jogging. Most dried fruits, including some of those found in muesli, are allowed on the Weight Control Plan. Dried apricots and prunes are the best options, since they both have a low GI value of 35; dried figs (GI of 40) are also acceptable. Dried fruits to avoid include raisins, sultanas, dried bananas, and dried coconut. Dried banana, in particular, is the worst dried fruit option for your waistline, as it has a high GI of 65.

FRUIT JUICE

Because commercially prepared fruit juices are high in sugar and low in fiber, they should be avoided at all costs. Even varieties that are labeled "freshly squeezed" may not be free from added sugar. What is more, many of these juices have the pulp removed, which is where all the fiber is. Although it is far healthier to eat a piece of fruit whole, you may drink homemade fruit juices, such as freshly squeezed orange juice, in moderation. It has a medium GI of 45 and will not contribute to weight gain. However, even freshly squeezed, homemade juices will be lower in fiber than their whole-fruit counterparts.

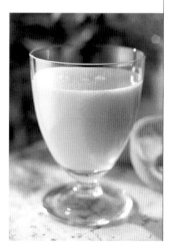

CANNED AND PRESERVED FRUITS

You may occasionally have low-GI fruit canned in water, with no sugar added. It is not an ideal fruit choice, since canned fruit is likely to contain artificial preservatives of some sort, and it contains less fiber than fresh and dried varieties. Fruits canned in syrup should be completely excluded because of the large amount of sugar added to make the syrup. In addition, fruit jams, sweetened with added sugar or grape juice, should be avoided throughout the diet. Replace these high-GI spreads with sugar-free fruit jams sweetened with fructose or artificial sweeteners.

"Most dried fruits, including some of those found in muesli, are allowed on the Weight Control Plan."

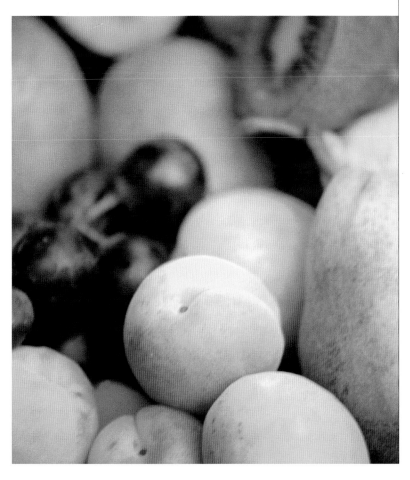

Left: kiwi, grapes, apricots, and pears are all acceptable fruits for weight maintenance.

On drinks

Even on the Weight Control Plan, caffeine and sugar can still upset your metabolism. This means that the basic rules for these beverages remain much the same as those for the Rapid Weight Loss Plan (*see pp70–71*). However, since your pancreas is not as sensitive as it once was, you can afford to be a little less rigorous in your application of the rules.

SOFT DRINKS

Avoid soft drinks, even on the Weight Control Plan. Regular varieties contain too much sugar and caffeine, and diet soft drinks contain artificial sweeteners that can have a similar effect to sugar on your blood-sugar levels (*see p52*). In place of synthetic soft drinks, try a tall glass of sparkling water with a twist of lemon or lime.

TEA AND COFFEE

Throughout the diet, avoid regular coffee and stick to the decaffeinated variety instead. Pure Arabica coffee is another option: it tastes just like regular coffee, but it is thought to be lower in caffeine. If you are a tea drinker, you may continue to drink weak black tea or herbal or fruit teas. That said, on the Weight Control Plan, you should have a higher tolerance threshold at which insulin is secreted, so consuming a little caffeine will not dramatically harm your metabolic equilibrium.

MILK

Avoid whole milk, since it is a complex food, consisting of proteins, saturated fats, and carbohydrates (lactose, or milk sugars). The watery part of milk (whey, which contains lactose) triggers the pancreas to produce insulin, which can trap the milk's saturated fat in the body for storage as fat tissue. Stick to skim milk instead, since it does not contain any saturated fat.

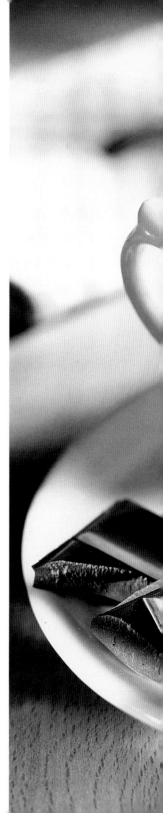

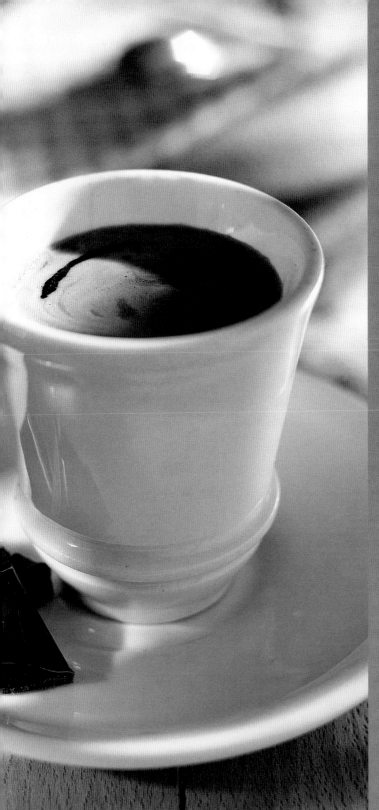

ESPRESSO

Few people know that real coffee—Italian espresso—is not very high in caffeine. This is because the high pressure of steam causes the ground coffee to release its magnificent flavor in concentrated form without releasing too much caffeine at the same time.

On the Weight Control Plan, when you have reached the goals you set for yourself at the start and your pancreas is functioning normally, you will be able to enjoy espresso, in moderation.

Allow yourself the occasional pleasure of taking a really good espresso at the end of your meal, along with a couple of squares of dark chocolate, if you wish.

Can I drink alcohol?

On the Weight Control Plan, you may drink alcohol in a moderate and controlled way. This is because your pancreas should have recovered its natural equilibrium, discharging the right amount of insulin to control the levels of glucose in the bloodstream. The golden rule on drinking alcohol while following the diet is to eat a protein-fat snack, such as cheese, before drinking anything.

Q How much wine and champagne can I drink?

On the Weight Control Plan, you may drink up to four 3.5-fl oz glasses of wine or champagne per day (but not all at once!) without destabilizing your metabolism. If the GI of your meal has not exceeded 50, then feel free to indulge in a couple of glasses. As on the Rapid Weight Loss Plan (*see pp72–73*), never drink on an empty stomach and always choose red wine, dry white wine, or good-quality champagne.

Q What about beer?

You may drink 12-fl oz of beer with food per main meal (i.e. lunch and dinner) on the Weight Control Plan without gaining weight. However, remember that beer is high in sugar, and it is easily converted into fat reserves. As on the Rapid Weight Loss Plan, you must refrain from drinking beer between meals. If you really cannot resist, approach the situation as you would any other discrepancy. That is, drink a couple of pints of the very best beer on offer at your favorite pub—but never do it on an empty stomach!

Q Can I have apéritifs?

Yes, so long as you indulge in moderation and eat a protein-fat snack first. Choose a high-quality red wine or champagne rather than a high-proof alcohol, such as vodka. The effects will be less serious, since the amount of alcohol contained in a glass of spirits is roughly equivalent to three or four glasses of red wine or champagne. If you must have a spirit-based apéritif, drink it neat (or mixed with water) and limit yourself to one.

Q Are after-dinner drinks acceptable?

If your meal has been accompanied by one small 3.5-fl oz glass of wine, a small quantity of cognac or sherry at the end will not have a catastrophic effect. However, if you drink a glass of cognac that rivals the size of a swimming pool, I would prefer not to be held responsible for the results—particularly if you have also consumed four or five glasses of wine during the course of your meal. Remember, though, that a generous glass of spirits is equivalent to about three or four glasses of wine.

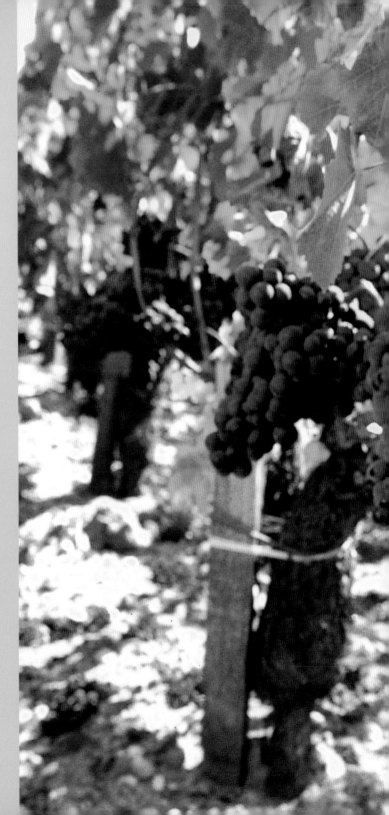

BENEFITS OF WINE

Many scientific studies
have shown that wine, particularly
red wine, has medicinal and
protective properties. The beneficial
effect of wine is due mainly to its
powerful antioxidants, which offer
valuable protection against by-
products of the metabolic process.
When consumed in moderate
amounts, the antioxidants in wine
may prevent the development of
some cancers, cardiovascular
disease, and even Alzheimer's
disease. In addition, wine may
improve the way your pancreas
responds to glucose in the
bloodstream, which helps to reduce
hyperinsulinism.

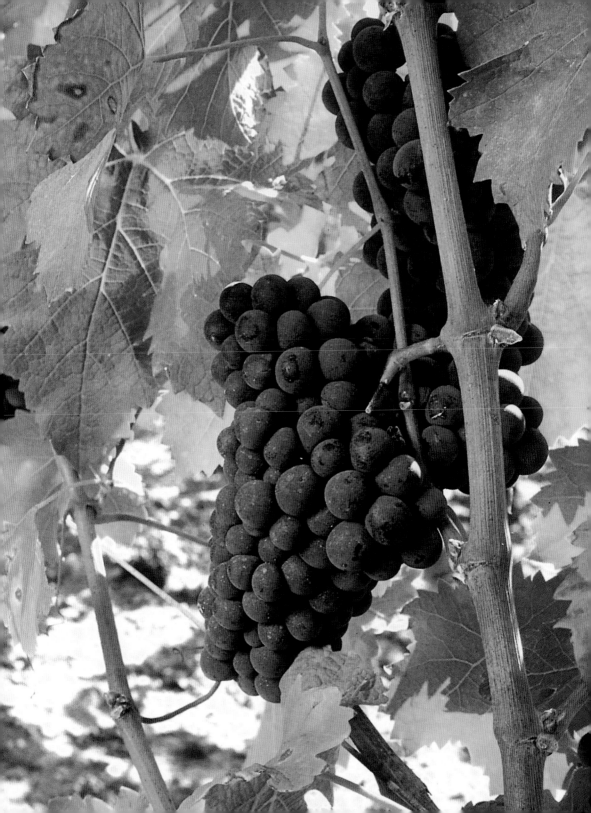

weight control

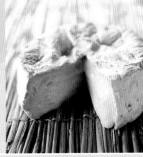

digested chapter

_____ **maintain your weight** and the health of your pancreas with the Weight Control Plan.

_____ **implement weight control** rules gradually, over several months, to avoid overburdening your pancreas. The Weight Control Plan should be viewed as a flexible extension of the Rapid Weight Loss Plan.

_____ **eat carbohydrates with a GI up to 50** without fear of gaining weight or destabilizing your pancreas.

_____ **have any protein or fat** you want with carbohydrates that have a GI of 50 or below. Flexibility is the hallmark of this plan, and there are no restrictive meal options for lunches and dinners.

KEY POINTS TO REMEMBER

use the AGI to eat the occasional carbohydrate with a GI slightly higher than 50, so long as you implement the AGI principle (*see pp112–14*), and eat it with high-fiber, low-GI vegetables.

you can drink wine, up to four 3.5-fl oz glasses, or two 12-fl oz bottles of beer, per day (but never on an empty stomach). You can also enjoy the occasional espresso, if you wish.

enjoy whole grain bread for breakfast and in the form of a snack called the Sandwich à la Montignac (*see pp144–45*). However, this is meant to be a snack, and bread (even good bread) should not be eaten at any other time of the day.

you may have two planned high–GI treats called discrepancies per month without fear of gaining weight (*see pp116–17*). If possible, try to choose a treat with a low carbohydrate concentration (*see p115*), and eat some low-GI, healthy carbohydrates first; then eat virtuously for the rest of the meal and the day.

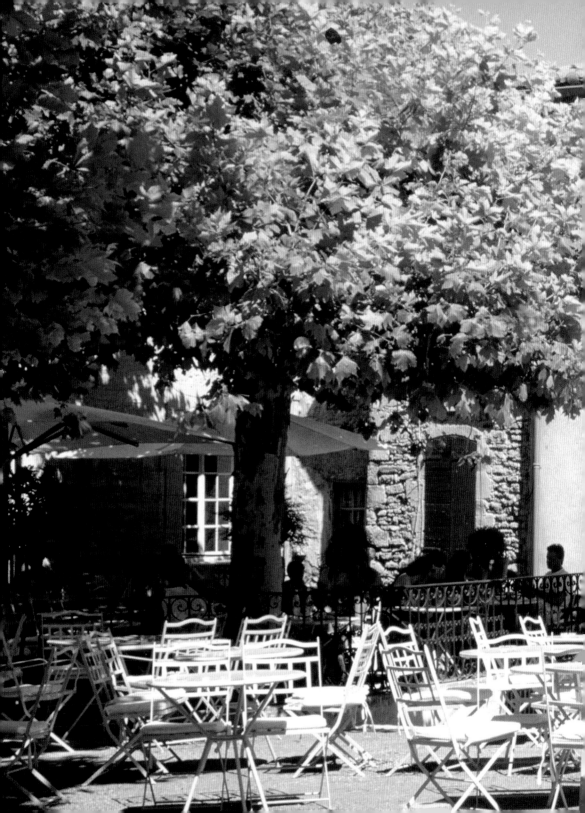

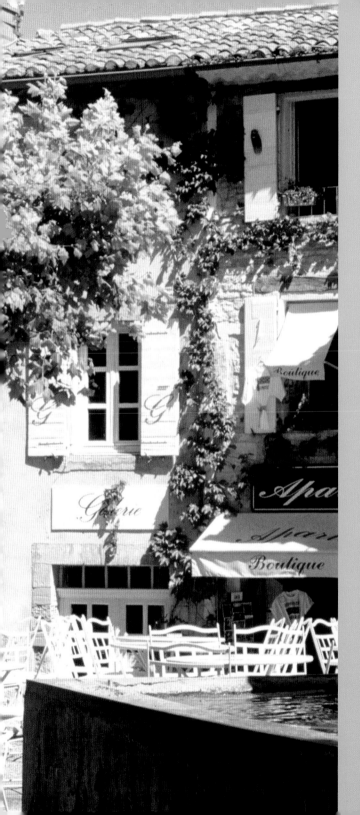

WEIGHT CONTROL: MEAL OPTIONS

On breakfast

Breakfast on the diet is a hearty meal that will not contribute to weight gain. On the Weight Control Plan (as on the Rapid Weight Loss Plan), there are two possible breakfast options: the carbohydrate–protein meal, which is built around good carbohydrates and a low or nonfat protein source, and the protein–fat breakfast, which is high in protein and saturated fats and free from carbohydrates. The carbohydrate–protein breakfast is still the healthier option of the two, and it should be eaten at least five days a week.

OPTION 1 carbohydrate–protein breakfast

The carbohydrate–protein breakfast from the Rapid Weight Loss Plan (*see pp80–81*) should be your staple breakfast on the Weight Control Plan. It contains very little saturated fat, a low or nonfat protein, and a

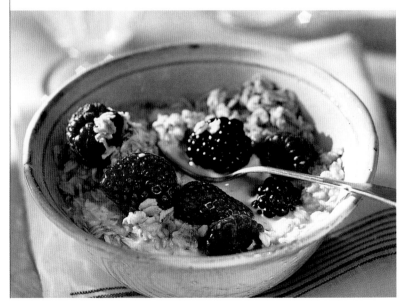

Right: *oat clusters with skim milk and fresh berries is an ideal carbohydrate-protein breakfast.*

high-fiber, low-GI carbohydrate. It may also include some low-GI fruit, if you wish. By combining acceptable carbohydrate and protein elements (*see below*), you can create such a diverse range of healthy and delicious breakfasts that it is unlikely that you will ever tire of this meal option.

For your carbohydrate element, look for foods that are rich in fiber and low in sugar. Some good examples of acceptable carbohydrate options include whole grain bread, rye bread, bread made with unrefined organic flour, sugarfree rice cakes, or sugarfree whole grain cereal, such as oat clusters. If, after about three months on the Weight Control Plan, you have grown tired of spreading your toast with sugar-free jam or jelly, you may use a light margarine instead.

For your protein element, choose protein-rich foods that are very low in, or completely free from, saturated fat. Skim milk or nonfat varieties of natural yogurt, cream cheese, cheese, and cottage cheese, are all good protein options. If you have a sweet tooth, you can add a little sugarfree jam to your yogurt or cream cheese.

OPTION 2   protein–fat breakfast

The protein-fat meal is an ideal choice for a relaxed, indulgent weekend breakfast. It consists of proteins and saturated fats, and should be completely free from carbohydrates. However, its high saturated fat content means this meal should be eaten no more than twice a week.

The protein portion of this meal can be ham, fish, cheese, or eggs. Eggs can be scrambled, boiled, fried, or made into an omelette. Scrambled eggs and sausage make a perfect protein-fat meal that will keep you feeling satisfied until lunch. (*For more options, see pp82–83.*) You can use fats such as butter in the preparation of this meal, and you can also have high-fat foods such as bacon with it. Eat as much as you like, so long as your breakfast does not include any carbohydrates with a GI higher than 35.

Because this breakfast is very high in fat, it is essential to balance this meal throughout the day by selecting foods for lunch and dinner that are rich in good carbohydrates and low in saturated fats.

"The protein-fat meal is an ideal choice for a relaxed, indulgent weekend breakfast."

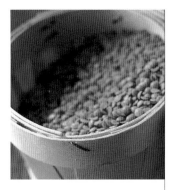

CARBOHYDRATES AND THE GI

An enormous range of carbohydrates is open to you on the Weight Control Plan. Eat whatever type you like with any type of protein or fat, so long as the carbohydrate has a GI of 50 or below. Good carbohydrates include lentils, pasta (cooked *al dente*), brown rice, wild rice, and sweet potatoes. However, it is a good idea to include some high-fiber, very low-GI vegetables in your meal, since they tend to be richer in vitamins than foods such as spaghetti and brown rice. The high levels of fiber they contain will also bring down the AGI (*see pp112–14*) of your meal.

Right, opposite: try lean roast beef, grilled mushrooms, and broccoli for a hearty Weight Control lunch.

On lunch

Lunch on the Weight Control Plan is a far more flexible affair than it was on the Rapid Weight Loss Plan, since there are no longer protein-fat or high-fiber carbohydrate meal options. There is simply one golden rule, and that is to keep the GI of your entire meal at or below 50. Do this, and you will maintain your weight and your healthy pancreas.

Have a filling lunch

The Weight Control lunch may consist of a soup, salad, side dish, and a main dish. You may also have wine or beer and a Montignac-approved dessert, if you wish (*for dessert options, see pp140–41*). Eat as much as you like, as this meal should be filling enough to keep you going until dinner. Your lunch should be made up of carbohydrates with a GI of 50 or below, some fat, and some protein in the form of meat, chicken, fish, tofu, or eggs. Eat any type of carbohydrate you like, so long as it has a GI of 50 or below. Do not skimp on very low-GI vegetables. They contain valuable nutrients that reduce the AGI (*see box, left*) of your meal.

Balance and moderation is key

The weight control lunch may include carbohydrates such as pasta (cooked *al dente*) or brown rice, if you wish. You can even prepare your food with oil or cream, within reason; do not drown your salad in oil or douse everything in cream. There are no restrictions on the type or amount of protein you choose, but it should always be prepared without breadcrumbs or flour. For a balanced diet, aim to eat a wide variety of protein-rich foods, such as fish, poultry, meat, and eggs.

Saturated fats (found in fatty meats and cream) should still be eaten in moderation, since they can contribute to cardiovascular disease. Trim any visible fat from your meat, and whenever possible, use unsaturated, good fats such as olive oil in place of saturated varieties.

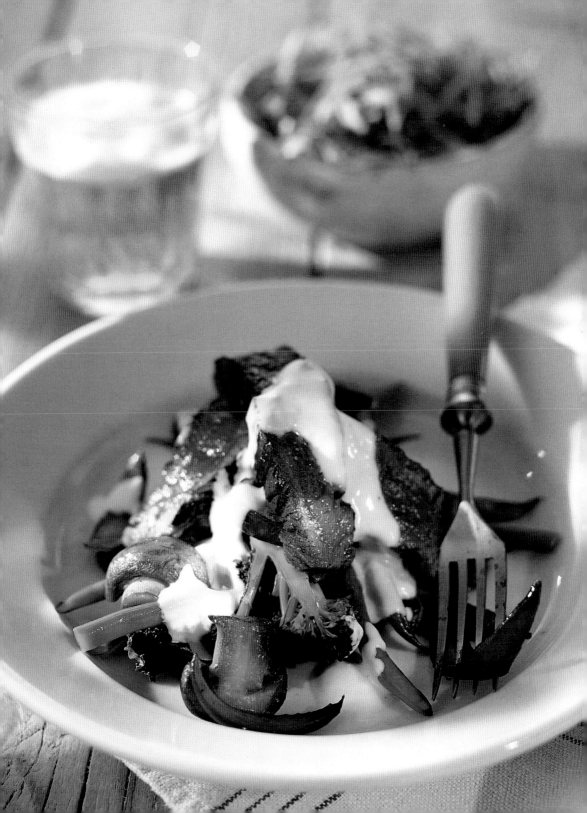

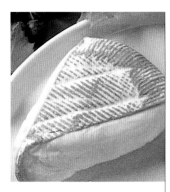

CHEESE

One of the great things about the Weight Control Plan is that you may eat cheese for dessert following any lunch or dinner. (On the Rapid Weight Loss Plan, you were advised not to eat regular cheese following a high-fiber carbohydrate meal.) The reason for this new flexibility is that your pancreas should be functioning normally on this plan. In other words, after eating carbohydrates with a GI of up to 50, your pancreas will not secrete an excess of insulin, and it will therefore not trap and store the saturated fat contained in the cheese.

On dessert

This section is very dear to me since I have a sweet tooth and am, by nature, a great lover of desserts at the end of a meal. As you might expect, all the desserts permitted on the Rapid Weight Loss Plan are also allowed on the Weight Control Plan. This plan is quite relaxed about desserts, provided you eat only foods with a GI of 50 or below. Luckily, this encompasses plenty of delicious options.

Nouvelle pâtisserie

Alongside the desserts you were allowed on the Rapid Weight Loss Plan (*see pp90–91*)—fresh and cooked fruit, low and nonfat cream cheese and natural yogurt, dark chocolate (70 percent cocoa), and cheese (*see box, left*)—you can also indulge in "nouvelle pâtisserie" (the nouvelle cuisine of desserts) on occasion. Just as nouvelle cuisine sauces seldom contain flour, nouvelle pâtisserie, especially the mousses, are made with very little sugar and hardly any flour.

French desserts

Perhaps I may be forgiven for claiming that French pastries are currently the best in the world for their originality, their beauty, their natural flavors and, above all, their lightness. Within the framework of this eating method, you are allowed to indulge in these delicacies throughout the Weight Control Plan. If you love pastries, try to eat only the lightest ones, which are, by the way, also the best ones. Those containing the least sugar and flour are most compatible with the diet's eating principles. Chocolate mousses made from dark bitter chocolate have few carbohydrates, and are particularly tasty.

For home chefs, the recipe for Raspberry and chocolate mousse (*see p237*) is delicious. It contains very few carbohydrates, and has a very low GI value. It can be eaten freely on the Weight Control Plan, and also occasionally on the Rapid Weight Loss Plan.

If you prefer cake, confine yourself to the very best chocolate cakes available. For example, a bitter chocolate fondant requires very little flour for a large cake. No sugar is added. The small amount of sugar in the chocolate is enough to make this cake an epicurean delicacy, one that will cause only a slight upset in your diet.

For those of you who like to create your own desserts from scratch, the Chocolate cake recipe in the back of this book is rich and decadent, but it contains no flour or added sugar at all (*see pp232–33 and below*). It derives its sweetness only from the dark chocolate it contains. It is therefore acceptable to eat for dessert on the Weight Control Plan.

In fact, none of the desserts in the recipe section at the back of this book (*see pp232–37*) have high GI values, and all of them are acceptable for both plans on the diet. To put it in perspective, almost any dessert you choose (from this book or your favorite restaurant) will cause less damage to your system than one horrible white potato.

"If you love pastries, try to eat only the lightest ones, which are, by the way, also the best ones."

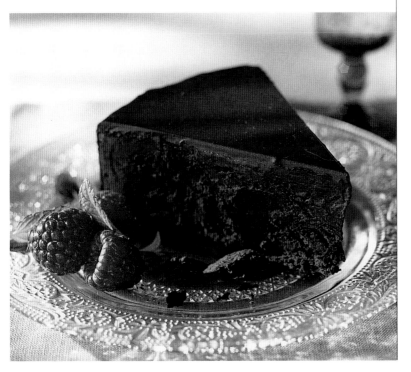

Left: Montignac's Chocolate cake (see pp232–33) is a delicious, low-GI dessert.

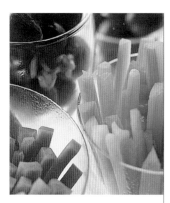

CARBOHYDRATES AND THE GI

As with lunch, you can eat whatever type of carbohydrate you want, so long as it has a GI of 50 or below. This might include unrefined Basmati rice, brown rice, spaghetti cooked *al dente*, chickpeas, kidney beans, or lentils. Do not skimp on high-fiber, very low-GI vegetables, since they provide a wide range of nutrients and the fiber they contain will bring down the AGI of your meal (*see pp112–14*) .

Right, opposite: Fresh cod and prosciutto rolls (see pp204–205) makes a healthy Weight Control dinner.

On dinner

The Weight Control dinner is very similar to the Weight Control lunch. This plan does not include protein-fat and high-fiber carbohydrate meal options—there is only one firm rule, and that is to eat carbohydrates with a GI of 50 or below. The only real difference between lunch and dinner is that your dinner should be lighter than your lunch.

Have a light dinner

Since most people's activity levels are lowest in the evening, fats eaten at night are more easily stored as body fat. Dinner should, therefore, be your lightest meal of the day. It should contain less fat and more vegetables than lunch, and if you want to have protein in the evening, it is preferable to choose fish or lean meats instead of fatty cuts. Fresh cod and prosciutto rolls (*see recipe on pp204–205*), served with salad and red wine, is an excellent example of a Weight Control dinner.

Like lunch, the Weight Control dinner may consist of a soup, salad, side dish, main dish, and dessert (*for Weight Control dessert options, see pp140–41*). To drink, you can have red wine, white wine, or beer, if you wish. Your dinner may include carbohydrates with a GI of 50 or below, as well as fats and protein in the form of lean meat, poultry, fish, tofu, or eggs. Take the time to enjoy each mouthful. Eat until you are full, but listen to your body and try not to overeat.

Fat and protein

Prepare your carbohydrates and proteins with any type of oil or fat you prefer, but try to use less of it than you did for your lunch. Remember, your body does not need fat in the evening, and it could be stored as body fat while you sleep. When choosing a protein, you should favor lean cuts of meat, removing any visible fat. Eggs, and especially fish, are also good options. Even fatty fish is fine because the kind of oil it contains will almost never be converted to fat.

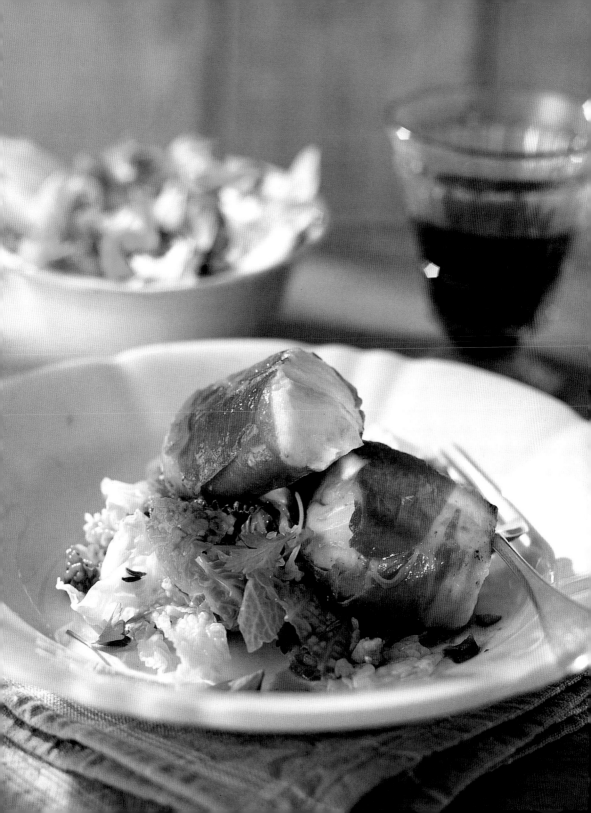

On snacks

Your meals should be hearty enough to keep you going, but if you feel the need for a snack, by all means have one. However, you should never reach for cookies or potato chips to stave off hunger pangs. For weight maintenance, the key to snacking lies in choosing healthful foods with a GI no higher than 50. The suggestions below are good snack options that will not destabilize your pancreas or cause you to gain weight.

Quick snacks

All of the very low-GI snack foods allowed while following the Rapid Weight Loss Plan are also permitted on the Weight Control Plan (*see pp98–99*). Snack on a handful of nuts, such as almonds, hazelnuts, or walnuts, or on a low-fat, sugarfree yogurt drink. You could even have a snack consisting only of fruit—eat as much as you like, so long as its GI value is 50 or below.

Alternatively, you could always stop at a delicatessen counter and order some boiled eggs or sliced meats and cheeses and eat them on their own, without bread or crackers. The proteins and fats these foods contain should keep you full for a few hours without increasing your blood-sugar levels and eliciting an insulin response.

Prepared snacks

If you like to plan ahead, you could prepare a wide variety of chopped raw vegetables such as carrots, tomatoes, and peppers, lean meats such as turkey or ham, and enjoy them with some cheese, such as cheddar, gruyère, or brie.

You could even throw together a salad niçoise to snack on (made with lettuce, boiled egg, tuna, tomatoes, anchovies, and black olives, drizzled with lemon juice and olive oil). If you prepare your snack ahead of time and carry it with you in a sealed container, you can avoid hunger attacks, and snack sensibly regardless of where you are.

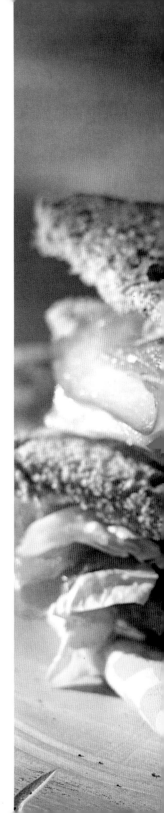

SANDWICH À LA MONTIGNAC

Snacks on the Weight Control plan can include bread in the form of the sandwich à la Montignac. Always use whole-wheat or rye bread, and toast it to slightly reduce its GI value. Between your two slices of bread you can have lean protein and any carbohydrate you like, provided it has a GI of 35 or below. However, you must avoid having any fats with it, except perhaps a little olive oil. One caveat: this sandwich is meant to be a light snack, eaten on an empty stomach. Filling suggestions include:

- **fish,** such as herring, tuna, and smoked salmon

- **lean meats,** including skinless chicken and turkey

- **low-GI vegetables,** such as lettuce, mushrooms, cucumber, raw carrots, peppers, and onions

- **sugar-free mustard** or horseradish

- **low-GI legumes,** including chickpeas and lentils

- **low-fat dairy products,** such as fat-free natural yogurt and low-fat cheese

weight control

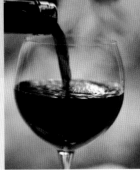

socializing

be demanding when dining at restaurants. Request that your meal be prepared without flour. It is always more effective to tell your waiter that you are allergic to flour than to say you are on a diet.

at dinner parties wait as long as possible into the meal before drinking any alcohol. Choose red wine if you can, pair it with some cheese, and drink no more than absolutely necessary.

if served pâté on toast at a dinner party, you can eat the pâté, which is generally a protein-fat, and leave the toast discreetly on the side of your plate. No one will notice!

at cocktail parties it is easier than you might think to "lose" your drink somewhere in the room. Place your glass on a surface near someone with an empty glass, and see how long it is before your glass is absent-mindedly picked up by an appreciative party guest.

canapés are out of the question, since the base is usually composed of a bad carbohydrate. However, they often support a slice of salmon, sausage, or boiled egg. Simply disassemble the canapé and eat only the good carbohydrate, fat, or protein contained on top.

cunning tactics are not always required at cocktail parties. Remember, any type of cheese is a good snack option, as is ham or sausage. So, too, are the ubiquitous cocktail sausages, spiked through with a toothpick and ready to enjoy.

come prepared if you feel that you will not be able to resist the culinary delights offered at a party. Take the edge off your appetite by having a protein-fat snack before you leave home.

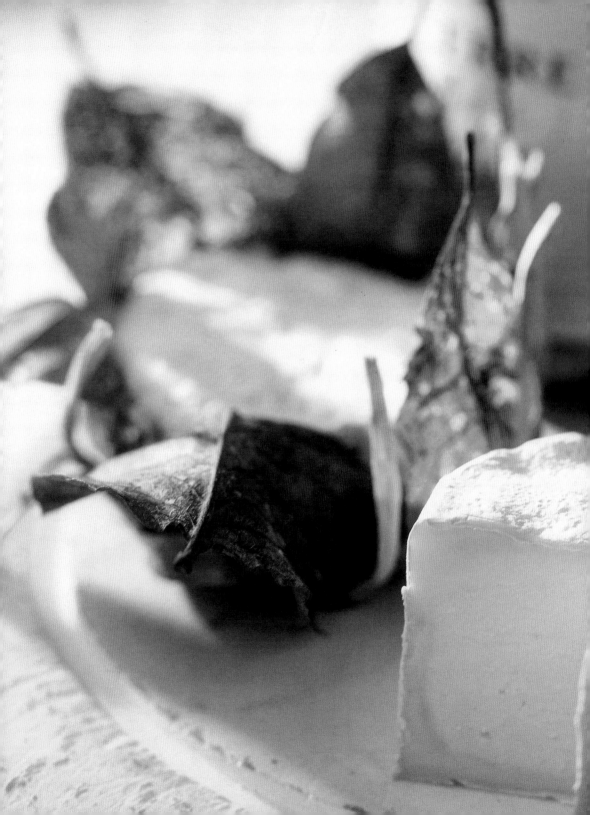

COCKTAIL TIPS

When at a cocktail party, always have a small protein-fat snack, such as cheese, before drinking any alcohol. When you drink on an empty stomach, the alcohol goes more rapidly into your bloodstream. This hinders weight loss and can even contribute to weight gain. In addition, if you must have an alcoholic apéritif, make it one of the following:

• **champagne** is the most acceptable alcoholic beverage to drink before a meal, but you must always have a protein-fat snack before taking your first sip. Never have more than one glass before you eat a meal.

• **dry red wine** is the next best type of alcohol you can choose. It is rich in antioxidants (see pp130–31; 246) and may help improve your tolerance to glucose. Again, limit yourself to only one glass before a meal, and always eat a protein-fat tidbit first.

• **dry white wine** is almost as good as dry red wine, but it lacks the powerful antioxidants found in red wine. Never have more than one glass with your protein-fat snack.

Weight Control menu plan

The Weight Control Plan is not a diet in the strict sense of the word. It is not concerned with limiting quantities of food or calories. Instead, it is a set of flexible guidelines for making good food choices. Use the following menu plan if you need some inspiration when planning your Weight Control meals and snacks.

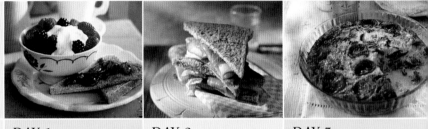

MEAL	DAY 1	DAY 2	DAY 3
Breakfast with herbal *or* fruit tea *or* decaffeinated coffee	• whole grain toast with sugar-free marmalade • low-fat natural yogurt with raspberries	• sugar-free oat clusters with skim milk and berries	• rice cakes topped with nonfat cheese and sliced apples
Lunch with two 3.5-fl oz glasses dry wine *or* one 12-fl oz glass beer	• vegetable soup, e.g. cream of asparagus soup • green salad • Linguini with ratatouille (*see p194*) • a few squares of dark chocolate	• vegetable soup, e.g. cream of cauliflower soup • broccoli sautéed with garlic and toasted walnuts • Tricolor rice with balsamic onions (*see p193*); grilled mushrooms • pears poached in red wine	• Cherry tomato soup with basil (*see pp160–61*) • Prawns à la pastis (*see p202*); brown rice with feta cheese • a few squares of dark chocolate
Snack (optional)	• hazelnuts and almonds	• Sandwich à la Montignac (*see pp144–45*)	• natural yogurt mixed with strawberries
Dinner with two 3.5-fl oz glasses dry wine *or* one 12-fl oz glass beer	• vegetable soup, e.g. mushroom soup • Pork chops in caper sauce (*see pp224–25*); spinach sautéed with garlic • Chocolate cake (*see pp232–33*)	• Soupe au vin blanc (*see p162*) • Cod on a bed of lentils (*see p198*); steamed artichokes • chopped apples mixed with cream cheese	• Red lentil soup with bacon (*see p164*) • green salad • Montignac Gruyère quiche (*see pp186–87*) • Raspberry and chocolate mousse (*see p237*)

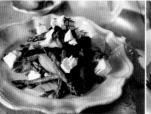 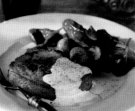 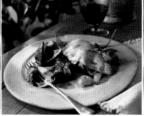 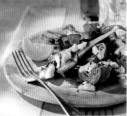

DAY 4	DAY 5	DAY 6	DAY 7
• toasted rye bread with nonfat cheese	• sugar-free oat clusters with skim milk and peaches	• omelette made with goat cheese and spinach • fried bacon	• poached eggs • grilled sausage
• Soupe au vin blanc (*see p162*) • Leek and asparagus salad (*see pp166–67*) • grilled salmon; baked sweet potato • peaches poached in wine	• Eggplant, basil, and cannellini soup (*see p163*) • lentils with sautéed mushrooms • Veal chops in Gorgonzola sauce (*see pp222–23*) • fresh figs and brie	• green salad • Chicken with figs (*see pp208–09*) • nonfat yogurt mixed with fresh raspberries	• Cherry tomato soup with basil (*see p160–61*) • green salad • Daube de boeuf (*see p219*) • peaches with cream cheese
• camembert and sliced apples	• selection of sliced meats	• Sandwich à la Montignac (*see pp144–45*)	• crudités with low-fat hummus dip
• Soupe au vin blanc (*see p162*) • roast turkey; brown rice with grilled zucchini • a few squares of dark chocolate	• vegetable soup, e.g. mushroom soup • Goat cheese salad (*see pp172–73*) • Coq au vin (*see pp210–11*) • natural yogurt with strawberries	• vegetable soup, e.g. tomato soup • sautéed artichoke hearts • Penne with capers and olives (*see p195*) • cream cheese with fresh strawberries	• vegetable soup, e.g. puréed cucumber soup • grilled salmon; Artichoke hearts with goat cheese (*see pp180–81*) • brie and apricots

Selection of good carbohydrates

Since carbohydrates are the only foods that contain sugar, GI values apply only to these foods. Fats and proteins (*see pp22–31*) contain very little, if any, sugar, so their impact on blood sugar levels are negligible. The following is a small selection of foods that can be eaten freely on the Weight Control Plan.

Avocados	10	Pecans	15
Almonds	15	Peppers (green)	15
Asparagus	15	Peppers (red)	15
Artichokes	15	Peppers (yellow)	15
Brazil nuts	15	Pumpkin seeds	15
Broccoli	15	Spinach	15
Brussels sprouts	15	Sunflower seeds	15
Cabbage (all kinds)	15	Walnuts	15
Cauliflower	15	Eggplant	20
Celery root	15	Fructose	20
Celery	15	Lemons	20
Zucchini	15	Limes	20
Cucumber	15	Chinese vermicelli (soybean variety)	22
Fennel	15	Beans, flageolet	25
Hazelnuts	15	Blackberries	25
Herbs	15	Cherries	25
Leeks	15	Dark chocolate (70 percent cocoa)	25
Lettuce (all kinds)	15	Lentils (green)	25
Mushrooms	15	Raspberries	25
Olives (all kinds)	15	Soybeans (cooked)	25
Onions (all kinds)	15	Split peas (yellow, cooked for 20 minutes)	25
Peanuts	15	Strawberries	25

Apples (fresh)	30	Peas (dried, cooked)	35
Apricots (fresh)	30	Peas (fresh, cooked)	35
Beans, fresh green or string beans	30	Plums	35
Carrots (raw)	30	Prunes	35
Chickpeas (cooked)	30	Quinoa	35
Fruit jam (sugarfree)	30	Satsumas	35
Garlic	30	Wild rice	35
Grapefuit	30	Black bread (German)	40
Lentils (brown)	30	Bread made from unrefined flour	40
Lentils (red)	30	Figs (dried)	40
Lentils (yellow)	30	Sorbet (sugarfree)	40
Milk (1% low-fat or skim)	30	Spaghetti, durum wheat (cooked *al dente*)	40
Mung beans (soaked and cooked for 20 minutes)	30	Spaghetti, whole wheat (cooked *al dente*)	40
Nectarines	30	Buckwheat	45
Peaches	30	Bulgur wheat (whole grain, cooked)	45
Pears	30	Grapes (all kinds)	45
Tomatoes	30	Rye (whole grain bread)	45
Apples (dried)	35	Orange juice (freshly squeezed)	45
Apricots (dried)	35	Whole grain bread with bran	45
Beans, broad (peeled and cooked)	35	Apple juice (fresh)	50
Beans, haricot	35	Crêpes/pancakes (made with buckwheat)	50
Figs (fresh)	35	Kiwi	50
Kidney beans	35	Rice (unrefined Basmati)	50
Natural yogurt	35	Rice (brown)	50
Oranges	35	Sweet potatoes	50

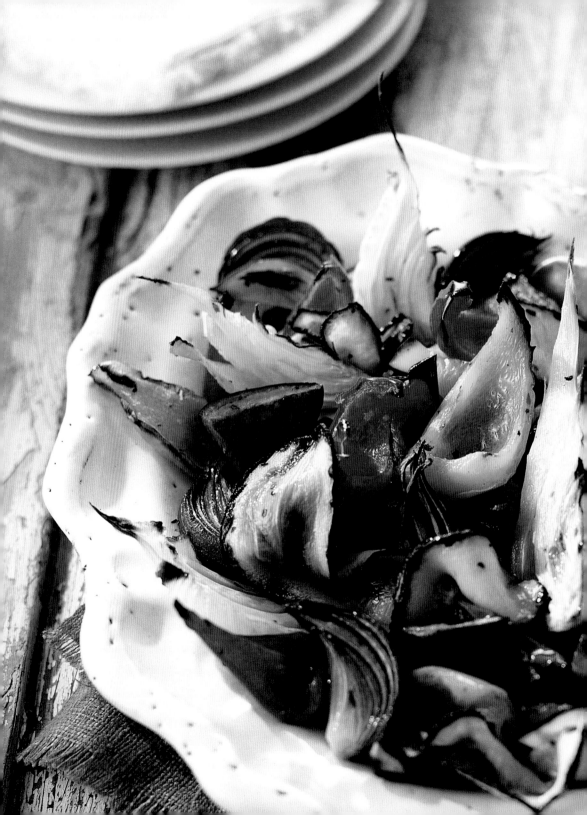

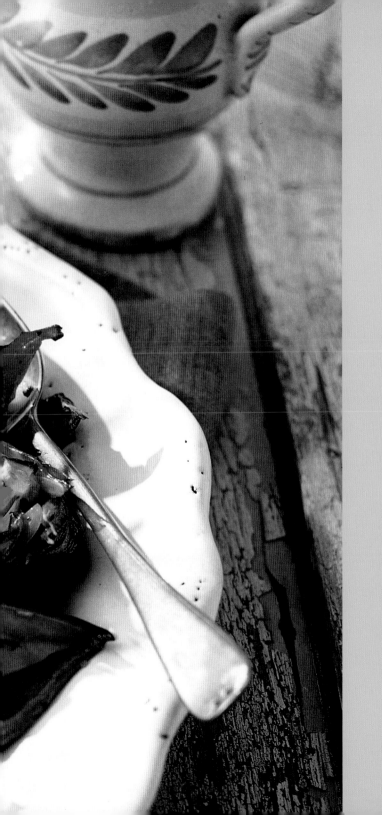

MONTIGNAC RECIPES

cooking

Montignac-style

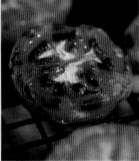

use low-GI carbohydrates when you cook, since they prevent weight gain. Good examples include vegetables, such as broccoli, cabbage, spinach, and zucchini; legumes including lentils and chickpeas (garbanzo beans); unrefined cereals and low-GI fruits.

eliminate high-GI carbohydrates when preparing meals. Foods to avoid include sugar, breadcrumbs, white flour, white potatoes, corn, white rice, and white pasta including ravioli, tortellini, and macaroni.

use good fats in your cooking whenever possible. These include olive oil, sunflower oil, walnut oil, pumpkin seed oil, goose fat, and duck fat (*for a more extensive list, see p41*).

eliminate bad fats from your cooking whenever possible. These include butter, coconut oil, palm oil, peanut oil, beef and pork drippings, lard, and hard, stick margarine (*for a more extensive list, see p41*).

avoid breadcrumbs and flour when cooking. Although any kind of cheese is acceptable, Parmesan makes a good substitute for breadcumbs. For sauces, replace white flour with puréed mushrooms or flour made from chickpeas, lentils, or soy beans.

add flavor to your cooking with dry red or white wine. They will not elicit a large insulin response or cause you to gain weight.

never use flour, butter, or sugar when making desserts. Instead, use sugar-free fruit purée, eggs, dark chocolate, fructose, and "flour" made from ground almonds or hazelnuts.

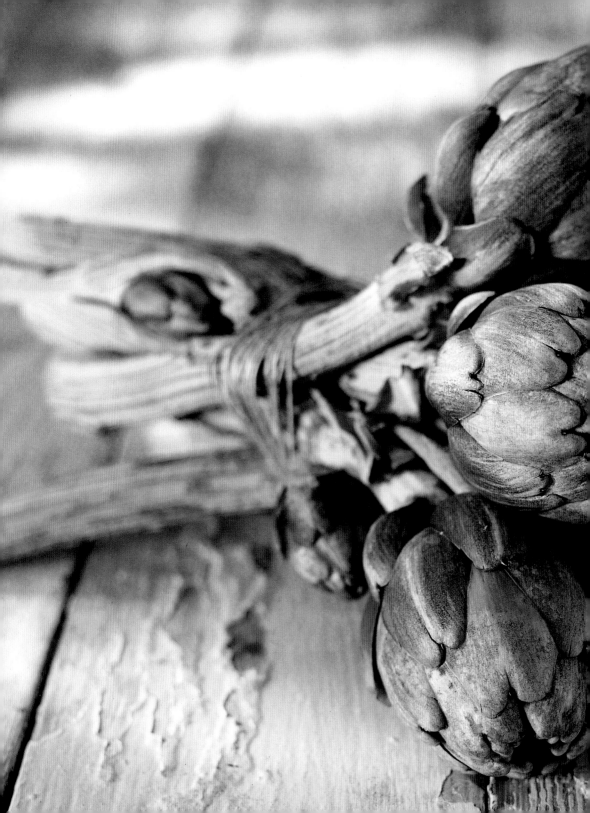

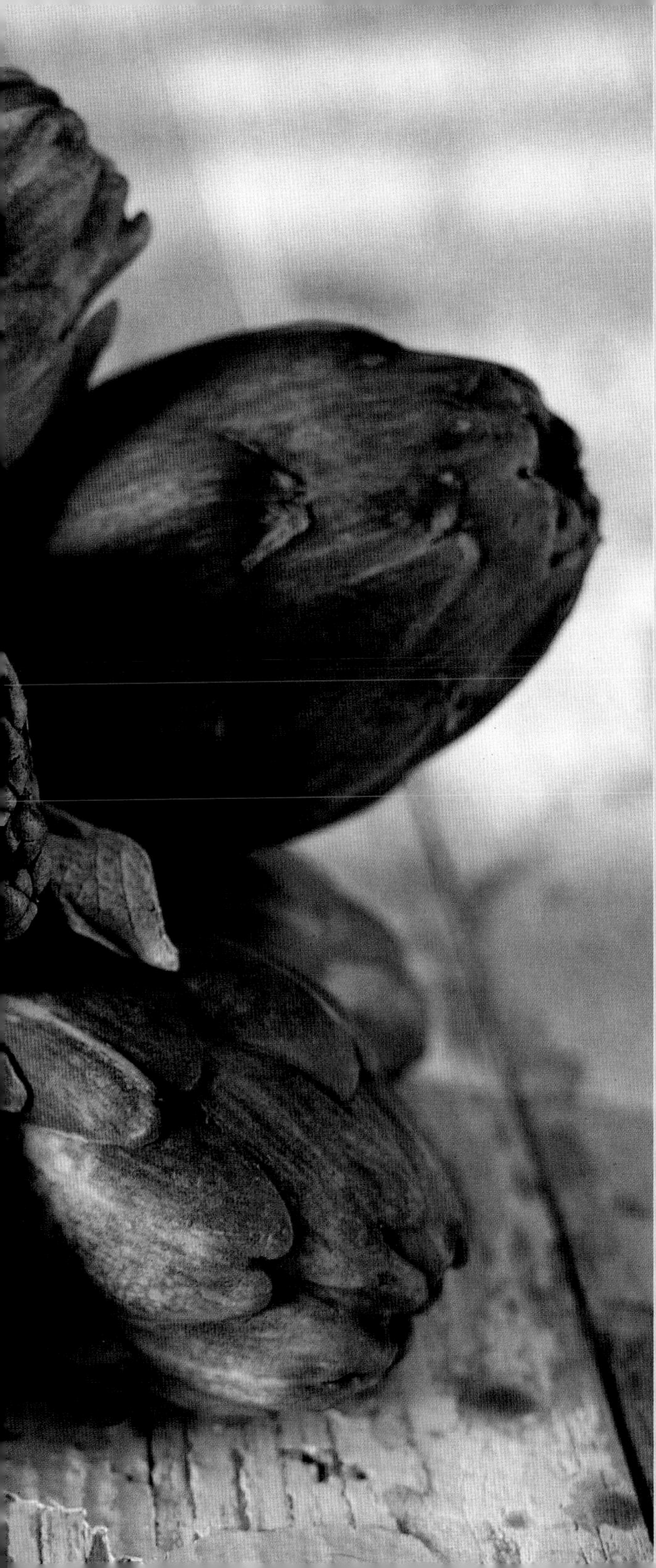

Starters

Montignac starters, which
include soups, salads, and
vegetable dishes, should
contain very low–GI
vegetables and be free
from high–GI
carbohydrates, such as
white potatoes and white
rice. Most of the recipes
in this section are
acceptable for both the
Rapid Weight Loss Plan
and the Weight Control
Plan except where noted.

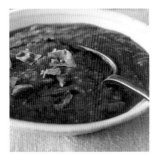

SERVES 4 TO 6

PREPARATION TIME
20 minutes

COOKING TIME
40 minutes

INGREDIENTS

1½ lb ripe cherry tomatoes

3 tbsp olive oil

1 tsp chopped fresh thyme

3 garlic cloves crushed
through a press or thinly
sliced

3 celery ribs, chopped

2 leeks (white and tender
green), well rinsed, chopped

2 white onions, chopped

1 tbsp tomato paste

¾ cup (lightly packed) fresh
basil leaves, stems reserved

1 (14½ oz) can diced
tomatoes, including juice

1 cup water or vegetable
stock

salt

ACCEPTABLE FOR
RAPID WEIGHT LOSS
and

WEIGHT CONTROL

Cherry tomato soup with basil

The deep, rich color of this flavorful soup is maintained by pushing it through a coarse sieve, rather than puréeing it in a blender or vegetable juicer. The latter methods incorporate air, making your soup more orange than red.

1   Preheat the oven to 500°F. Arrange the cherry tomatoes on a baking sheet and drizzle with 1½ tablespoons olive oil. Sprinkle with thyme and garlic, and toss to coat. Roast until tomatoes are softened but still hold their shape, 5 to 7 minutes. Set aside to cool.

2   Meanwhile, heat 1 tablespoon of oil in a large, heavy-bottomed saucepan or soup pot over medium heat. Stir in the celery, leeks, and onions. Cook, covered, until softened but not browned, 5 to 10 minutes. Stir in the tomato paste and the reserved basil stems.

3   Stir in chopped tomatoes with their juice, then add the cherry tomatoes. Pour in the water, reduce heat to low, and cook, uncovered, 20 minutes to blend flavors.

4   Press the soup through a coarse sieve or food mill, discarding the tomato skins and basil stems. Return mixture to the same pot, adding salt to taste, and reheat gently.

5   Serve the soup hot in warmed bowls. Tear the basil leaves into pieces and scatter over each serving; then drizzle with the remaining olive oil.

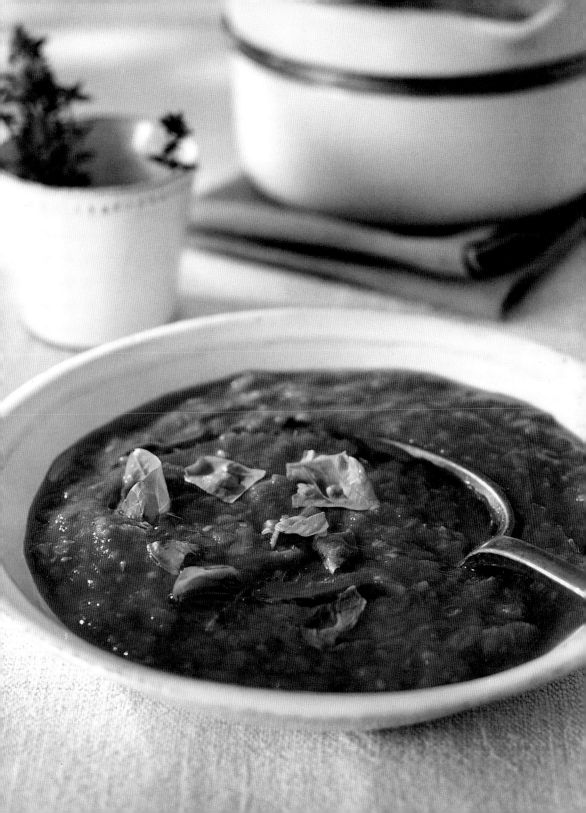

Soupe au vin blanc

SERVES 4 TO 6

PREPARATION TIME
10 minutes

COOKING TIME
20 minutes

INGREDIENTS
1 tbsp olive oil
6 shallots, finely chopped
1 lb button mushrooms, sliced
1½ cups dry white wine
3 tbsp tarragon vinegar
3½ cups good-quality white chicken stock (preferably homemade)
1 lb ground blanched almonds
2 cups heavy (whipping) cream
salt
3 tbsp chopped fresh tarragon

ACCEPTABLE FOR
RAPID WEIGHT LOSS
and
WEIGHT CONTROL

To keep the color of this soup as white as possible, either make your own white chicken stock without carrots, or purchase good-quality stock that is not too yellow.

1 In a large, heavy-bottomed saucepan, heat the oil over medium heat. Stir in the shallots and cook, covered, 3 to 5 minutes, or until the shallots are softened but not browned.

2 Add the mushrooms, wine, and tarragon vinegar. Cook uncovered, stirring, 5 minutes to blend flavors. Pour in the chicken stock and bring to a boil.

3 Whisk in the almonds. Cook, stirring occasionally, until mixture returns to a boil. (This will bring out the gluten in the almonds.) Whisk in the cream and return to a boil.

4 Skim off any foam that rises to the top. Reduce heat to low and add salt to taste. Stir in the tarragon.

5 Serve the soup hot in warmed bowls.

Eggplant, basil, and cannellini soup

SERVES 4 TO 6

PREPARATION TIME
30 minutes, plus 12 hours for soaking beans

COOKING TIME
2 hours

INGREDIENTS
1 cup (7 oz) cannellini beans, soaked overnight in enough water to cover by at least 2-in

6 large shallots, finely chopped

1 garlic head, cloves separated and finely chopped (about 3 tbsp)

3 large eggplant, halved lengthwise

salt

2 tbsp chopped fresh thyme

⅓ cup olive oil

3 bunches of fresh basil, about 2 cups lightly packed, leaves torn, plus extra, chopped, to serve

1½ cups dry white wine

5½ cups good-quality chicken stock (preferably homemade)

ACCEPTABLE FOR
RAPID WEIGHT LOSS
and

WEIGHT CONTROL

Don't be tempted to skimp on the fresh basil and thyme in this hearty soup. The herbs are the secret to lifting the flavors, as they soften the substance of the cannellini beans and eggplant.

1 Drain the cannellini beans and rinse with cold water. Turn into a heavy-bottomed saucepan and cover with fresh, cold water. Bring to a boil over high heat. Reduce heat to low and simmer partially covered up to 1½ hours, until just tender. Drain and set aside.

2 Preheat the oven to 500°F. Place the eggplant cut-side up on a baking sheet. Using a sharp knife, score the flesh in a crisscross pattern about 1½-inches deep, and season with salt. Sprinkle each with 1 teaspoon of garlic, scatter with thyme, and drizzle with half the olive oil. Roast 20 to 30 minutes, until tender. When cool enough to handle, peel off the skin and discard. Coarsely chop the flesh and set aside.

3 Add the remaining olive oil to a large, heavy-bottomed saucepan. Add the shallots and cook, covered, 3 to 5 minutes, or until softened but not browned. Add the remaining garlic, ⅔ of the cannellini beans, and the basil leaves. When the basil has wilted, pour in the wine and stock. Simmer 5 minutes to blend flavors.

4 In a food processor or blender, combine ⅓ of the eggplant flesh and ⅓ of the cannellini beans with the remaining soup. Process until a coarse purée forms. Return mixture and the remaining roasted eggplant, coarsely chopped, to the rest of the soup. Cook uncovered over medium heat, stirring occasionally, until heated through.

5 Serve hot in warmed bowls, with extra basil sprinkled on top.

Red lentil soup with bacon

SERVES 4 TO 6

PREPARATION TIME
30 minutes, plus 12 hours
for soaking beans

COOKING TIME
2½ hours

INGREDIENTS
½ cup dried chickpeas
(garbanzo beans), soaked
overnight in water to cover
by 2-in (or use 1 can
garbanzo beans, drained)

1 tbsp olive oil

¼ lb thick-sliced bacon, cut
crosswise, or pancetta, cut
into ½-in cubes

3 leeks (white and tender
green), well rinsed, coarsely
chopped

2 large onions, coarsely
chopped

3 celery ribs, coarsely
chopped

2 carrots, coarsely chopped

1 tbsp chopped fresh thyme
leaves

½ cup red lentils, picked over
and rinsed

2 qts water

salt

ACCEPTABLE FOR

WEIGHT CONTROL

The most time consuming part of making this rustic and robust soup is soaking the chickpeas, but canned may be used if you prefer. Remember not to add salt to the chickpeas while they are cooking, as it toughens their skins.

1   Drain the chickpeas in a colander and rinse with fresh water. Turn into a saucepan and cover well with fresh, cold water. Bring to a boil over high heat and simmer for 1 to 1½ hours, or until tender. Drain and set aside.

2   Heat the olive oil in a large, heavy-bottomed saucepan over medium-high heat. Add the bacon and cook, stirring occasionally, until nicely browned. Stir in the leeks, onions, celery, carrots, and thyme. Cook, covered, 3 to 5 minutes, until softened but not browned.

3   Add the lentils and chickpeas. Pour in the water and bring to a boil. Reduce heat to low and cook, uncovered, 45 minutes to blend flavors.

4   In a blender or food processor, working in batches, process the soup, pulsing the machine on and off to form a coarse purée. Reheat and taste, adding salt as needed.

5   Serve soup hot in warmed bowls.

Chicken salad with mustard dressing

SERVES 4

PREPARATION TIME
20 minutes

COOKING TIME
20 minutes

INGREDIENTS
2 boneless, skinless chicken breast halves, about 6 oz each

1 tbsp olive oil

salt

3 large carrots, cut into sticks ¼-in wide and 1-in long

6 medium celery ribs, cut into sticks ¼-in wide and 1-in long

⅓ cup mayonnaise

2 tbsp coarse-grain mustard

4 small hearts of romaine, separated into leaves

vinaigrette (see page 169)

ACCEPTABLE FOR
  RAPID WEIGHT LOSS
and

  WEIGHT CONTROL

The contrast of flavors and textures sets this chicken salad apart. Crisp lettuce is a delicious counterpoint to the creamy chicken, while the tangy mustard complements the lemon vinaigrette.

1 Preheat the oven to 300°F. Coat the chicken breasts with olive oil and season with salt. Place on a baking sheet and bake for 12 minutes. Turn the breasts over and bake 4 to 8 minutes longer, until the chicken is cooked through, but still juicy. Set aside 15 to 20 minutes to cool.

2 Slice chicken into strips and place in a bowl with the carrots, celery, onion, and parsley.

3 Add the mayonnaise and mustard, and toss gently to coat. Taste, adding more salt as needed.

4 Lay a few lettuce leaves flat on each of 4 salad plates and mound equal portions of chicken salad on top.

5 Drizzle each serving with 1 tablespoon of vinaigrette and serve.

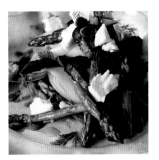

Leek and asparagus salad

The strong, earthy flavors of the leek, eggplant, and artichoke are enhanced by fragrant herbs and crisp pumpkin seeds. If you are unable to find pumpkinseed oil, substitute extra virgin olive oil for the finishing touch.

SERVES 4 TO 6

PREPARATION TIME
20 minutes

COOKING TIME
25 minutes

INGREDIENTS
1½ lb asparagus, cut into 3-in lengths

salt

olive oil

4 large eggplant, each quartered lengthwise and cut crosswise into cut into ½-in slices

8 leeks, (white and tender green) well rinsed, cut into ½-in rounds

1 (14 oz) can artichoke hearts, drained and halved

2 tbsp chopped fresh dill

2 tbsp chopped fresh chervil

½ cup hulled, roasted pumpkin seeds (pepitas)

1 cup feta cheese, diced or crumbled

pumpkinseed oil to finish

ACCEPTABLE FOR
RAPID WEIGHT LOSS
and

WEIGHT CONTROL

1 Heat 1 tablespoon olive oil in a large skillet over medium–high heat. Working in batches, add asparagus without crowding. Cook, stirring and tossing, until lightly charred on the outside and just barely tender, 3 to 5 minutes. Repeat with remaining asparagus, adding more oil only if needed. Remove from the pan and set aside to cool.

2 Season the eggplant with a pinch of salt and drizzle lightly with olive oil. In the same skillet and working in batches, heat 1 tablespoon olive oil over medium–high heat. Cook, stirring frequently, until eggplant is tender and lightly browned, about 15 minutes. Repeat with remaining eggplant, adding oil as needed. Remove from the pan and set aside to cool.

3 In the same skillet, heat another tablespoon of oil over medium–high heat. Add the leeks, stirring to coat. Season lightly with salt. Cook, covered, until softened and lightly browned at the edges, 3 to 5 minutes. Remove from the pan and drain in a colander while cooling.

4 In a large bowl, combine the asparagus, eggplant, and leeks. Sprinkle with the dill, chervil, and pumpkin seeds. Drizzle a little pumpkinseed oil on top and add in the feta. Toss gently to mix

5 This salad is best served at once. Serve at room temperature.

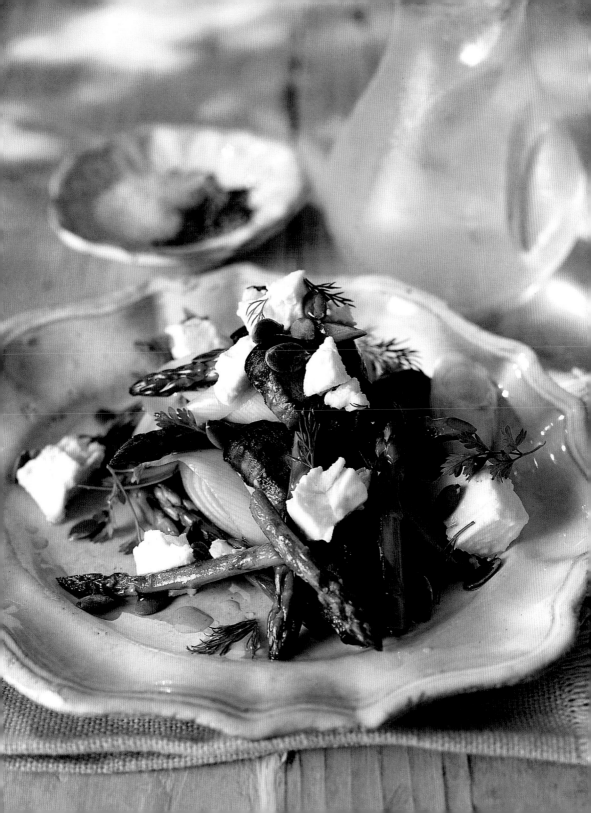

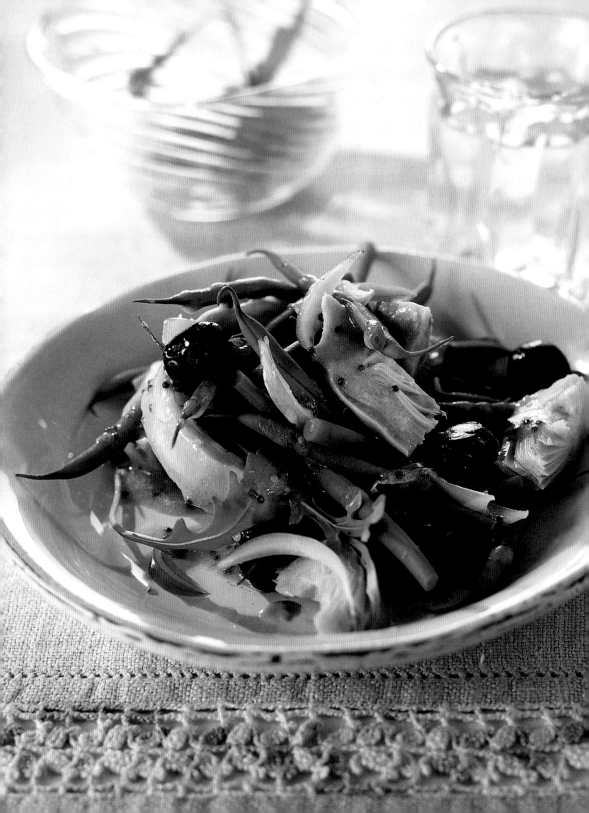

Green bean, artichoke, and arugula salad

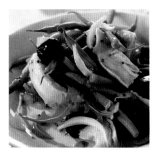

SERVES 4

PREPARATION TIME
20 minutes

COOKING TIME
25 minutes

INGREDIENTS
4 globe artichokes

2 lemons, halved

½ lb thin green beans or haricots vert, trimmed

3 (6 oz) cans marinated artichoke hearts, drained and halved

2 shallots, finely chopped

25 kalamata olives, pitted (about ½ cup)

8½ oz arugula

½ cup freshly grated Parmesan cheese

FOR THE VINAIGRETTE
1 tsp each lemon juice, white wine vinegar, Dijon mustard, and coarse-grain mustard

½ cup (4 fl oz) each olive oil and sunflower oil

salt

ACCEPTABLE FOR
  RAPID WEIGHT LOSS
and

  WEIGHT CONTROL

This deceptively simple assembly is rich with Mediterranean flavors. For best results, use the highest quality ingredients you are able to find.

1 Add lemon juice to a bowl of cold water; reserve the juiced halves. One by one, pull back artichoke leaves until they break off naturally. Continue until you reach the pale green "heart." Cut off tough ends from artichoke stems.

2 Cut hearts in half lengthwise and trim away any dark green bits. Scrape out the fuzzy choke with a spoon. Rub the cut parts with lemon halves as you work.

3 Add artichoke hearts to a pot of boiling salted water. Reduce heat to low and cook, covered, until tender, 10 to 15 minutes. Drain in a colander and set aside to cool.

4 In another pot of boiling water, cook green beans 2 to 3 minutes until crisp-tender. Drain and rinse with cold water.

5 Combine the green beans, cooked fresh and canned artichoke hearts, shallots, and olives in a bowl. Set aside.

6 To make the vinaigrette, whisk together the lemon juice, vinegar, and mustards. Slowly whisk in the oils. Salt to taste. Add enough vinaigrette to coat the vegetables.

7 Add arugula and toss gently to mix. Turn salad onto a serving platter. Sprinkle Parmesan over the top and serve.

SERVES 4

PREPARATION TIME
30 minutes

COOKING TIME
20 minutes

INGREDIENTS
3 slices crisp, cooked bacon, coarsely chopped

3 slices thick-cut bacon, cut crosswise into ¼-in pieces

1 cup vine-ripened cherry tomatoes, halved

4 oz Emmental or Jarlsberg cheese, diced (about 1 cup)

4 oz thin green beans or haricots vert, trimmed

8 black olives, pitted

8 green olives, pitted

8 oz mixed baby lettuces, such as lollo rosso, dandelion, frisée

walnut oil

freshly ground pepper

WALNUT DRESSING
4 tbsp red wine vinegar

3 tbsp sherry vinegar

2 tbsp Dijon mustard

⅔ cup sunflower oil

2½ tbsp walnut oil

pinch of salt

ACCEPTABLE FOR
  RAPID WEIGHT LOSS
and
  WEIGHT CONTROL

Mélange of salads

Walnut oil imparts a distinctive nutty flavor and aroma, so look for high-quality brands—often imported—sold in high-end supermarkets and delis.

1 Heat the oven to 475°F. Place the cooked bacon on a baking sheet and reheat until it becomes crisp again, 3 to 5 minutes. Drain on paper towels.

2 Meanwhile, cook the thick-cut bacon in a skillet over medium heat, turning frequently, until it is nicely browned, 5 to 10 minutes. Drain on paper towels.

3 Place the cherry tomatoes in a colander and sprinkle with salt. Toss gently. Let sit to drain off excess juice.

4 Bring a pot of salted water to a boil over high heat. Add green beans. When water returns to a boil, cook 2 to 3 minutes longer, or until beans are crisp-tender. Immediately drain in a colander. Rinse with cold water and drain again.

5 To make the walnut dressing, combine all the ingredients in a glass jar and shake well. (You can store any leftover dressing in the refrigerator for up to 4 weeks.)

6 In a large bowl, combine the bacon pieces and cubes, tomatoes, beans, cheese, and olives. Drizzle with walnut dressing to moisten. In a separate bowl, drizzle the salad greens with a little walnut oil. Add salt and freshly ground black pepper to taste.

7 To serve, alternately layer the bacon mixture and salad leaves in a serving bowl or on individual plates.

2-bean and tuna salad

Dry-roasting spices brings out their full potential, giving a more complex flavor than their pre-ground counterparts.

SERVES 4 TO 6

PREPARATION TIME
15 minutes

COOKING TIME
8 minutes

INGREDIENTS

¼ cup cumin seed

¼ cup coriander seed

¼ cup fennel seed

2 tsp hot red chili flakes

1 head of garlic, cloves separated and finely chopped (about ¼ cup)

olive oil

1 cup red wine vinegar

1 cup (8 oz) cherry tomatoes, quartered or halved

1¼ cups cooked flageolet, navy, or any other white beans, drained

4 small bell peppers, seeded and chopped, preferably mixed colors

2 small red onions, finely chopped

¼ lb thin green beans or haricots vert, trimmed

4 fresh red jalapeño chili peppers, seeded and finely chopped

1 tbsp chopped fresh basil

1 tbsp chopped fresh mint

3 (6 oz) cans chunk light tuna packed in oil, drained

ACCEPTABLE FOR

RAPID WEIGHT LOSS

and

WEIGHT CONTROL

1 Combine the cumin seed, coriander seed, fennel seed, and chili pepper flakes in a dry skillet. Cook over low heat until fragrant, about 30 seconds to 1 minute. Grind to a powder in an electric coffee mill or with a mortar and pestle.

2 Heat 1 tablespoon olive oil in a skillet over medium heat. Add the garlic and cook 1 minute to release the flavor. Add the ground spices, then pour in the red wine vinegar. Transfer everything to a stainless-steel bowl and let cool completely. (Recipe can be prepared in advance up to this point.)

3 Bring another pot of salted water to a boil over high heat. Add green beans. When water returns to a boil, cook 2 to 3 minutes longer, or until the beans are crisp-tender. Immediately drain in a colander. Rinse with cold water and drain again.

4 Place the flageolet beans, bell peppers, red onions, green beans, chili peppers, basil, and mint in a bowl. Add the tuna and gently toss.

5 Add a few tablespoons of the vinegar spice mix and 2 tablespoons olive oil. Taste, adding salt and more vinegar-spice as desired. Add cherry tomatoes, tossing gently. Serve in a large bowl.

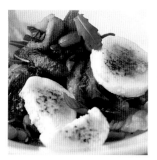

Goat cheese salad

Smoky roasted peppers, creamy goat cheese, and peppery arugula—all dressed with a lemon vinaigrette enlivened by fresh herbs—combine to make a light but satisfying salad perfect for a spring or summer lunch.

SERVES 4

PREPARATION TIME
30 minutes

COOKING TIME
25 minutes

INGREDIENTS
8 oz baby lima beans
4 large yellow peppers
6 tbsp olive oil plus extra for drizzling
4 large ripe tomatoes
1 tbsp chopped fresh basil
salt
1 tbsp chopped fresh mint
juice of ½ lemon
½ lb arugula
5-7 oz soft goat cheese, cut into ½-in slices

ACCEPTABLE FOR
 RAPID WEIGHT LOSS
and

 WEIGHT CONTROL

1 Preheat the oven to 500°F. Cut the peppers in half lengthwise and remove the stems and seeds. Place them cut-side down on a baking sheet. Roast 20 minutes, or until the skins are charred. Do not turn off the oven. Remove and set aside. When cool enough to handle, rub off the skins. Cut peppers into ½-inch strips.

2 To blanch the tomatoes, plunge into boiling salted water for 15 to 30 seconds, then plunge into a bowl of ice cold water. Peel off and discard the skin, slice the flesh into quarters, and remove the seeds. Slice the flesh into ¼-inch strips. In a large bowl, combine the peppers, tomatoes, lima beans, and arugula.

3 In a small bowl, whisk together the 6 tablespoons olive oil, a pinch of salt, basil, mint, and lemon juice. Add to the salad, tossing gently to mix. Divide salad among 4 plates.

4 Place the goat cheese on a greased baking sheet. Bake until cheese is heated through, but still holds its shape, 1 to 2 minutes. Top each salad with the warm goat cheese and serve at once.

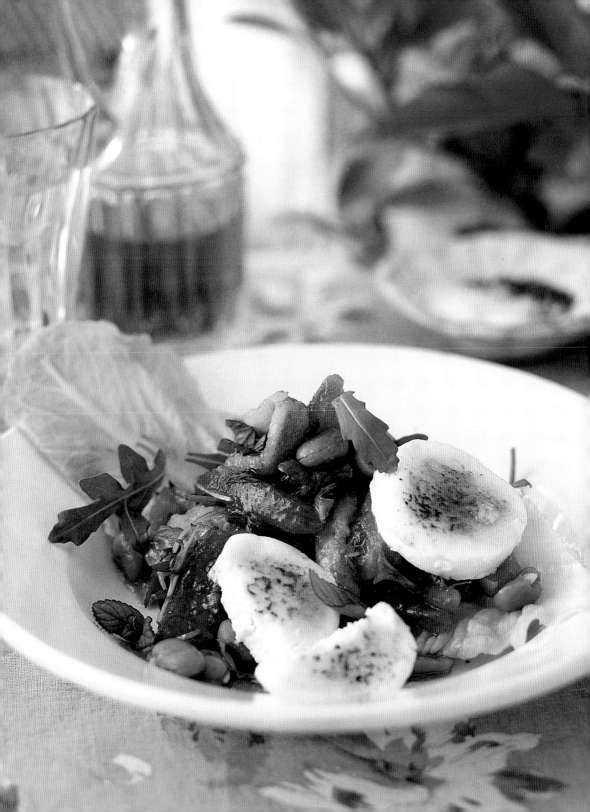

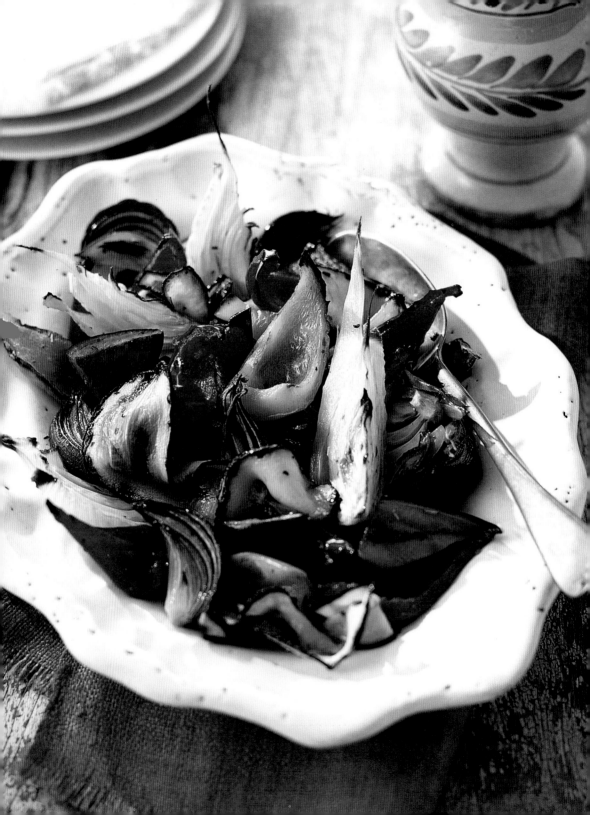

Mediterranean oven-roasted vegetables

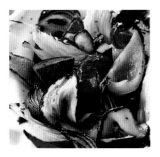

There is a world of difference between genuine herbes de Provence and the pale imitation often found on supermarket shelves. Take the time to search out the best brand you can find.

SERVES 4 TO 6

PREPARATION TIME
30 minutes

COOKING TIME
45 minutes

INGREDIENTS
3 small eggplant, quartered lengthwise and cut into ½-in thick slices

olive oil

salt

4 yellow peppers, seeded and cut into large chunks

4 red peppers, seeded and cut into large chunks

2 tbsp herbes de Provence

3 tbsp garlic purée

2 medium fennel bulbs, cut into ½-in wedges

2 medium red onions, cut into ½-in wedges

2 large zucchini, sliced lengthwise, ¼-in thick

ACCEPTABLE FOR
  RAPID WEIGHT LOSS
and

  WEIGHT CONTROL

1   Preheat the oven to 500°F. Place the eggplant on a baking sheet with olive oil, and season with salt. Roast in the oven for 15 to 20 minutes, or until browned and tender. Remove from the oven and let cool. Reduce the oven temperature to 425°F.

2   Place the yellow and red peppers on a baking sheet, drizzle with a little olive oil, and sprinkle with salt, half of the herbes de Provence, and the garlic purée. Roast 10 minutes. Remove from the oven, place in a colander to strain off juices, and let cool. Keep the oven at the same temperature.

3   Place the fennel, onions, and zucchini on a baking sheet, and drizzle with olive oil, salt, and the remaining herbes de Provence. Roast 8 minutes, or until the fennel is just tender and the onion is lightly browned. (If desired, roast these vegetables at the same time as the peppers—just remember to take them out after 8 minutes.) Let cool.

4   In a large bowl, combine all the vegetables. Toss gently to mix. Serve at room temperature.

Rainbow lentils

SERVES 4

PREPARATION TIME
10 minutes

COOKING TIME
20 minutes

INGREDIENTS
½ cup (4 oz) green lentils,
picked over and rinsed

½ cup (4 oz) red lentils,
picked over and rinsed

½ cup (4 oz) brown lentils,
picked over and rinsed

½ cup (4 oz) yellow lentils,
picked over and rinsed,

olive oil

fine sea salt

ACCEPTABLE FOR
RAPID WEIGHT LOSS
and

WEIGHT CONTROL

This straightforward side dish is enhanced by simply adding a little sea salt and olive oil just before serving. It is important not to add salt to the lentils at the start of cooking, because this will toughen them.

1   To cook the lentils, place in separate small saucepans and cover each with about 1½-in of cold water. Bring the green, red, and brown lentils to a boil over medium-high heat. Reduce heat to low and cook 10 to 20 minutes, until barely tender. The yellow lentils will take about 5 minutes to cook and need only be brought to a boil.

2   Season with salt and cook 3 minutes longer, until tender. Place in a sieve, rinse with cold water, and drain well.

3   Combine all the lentils in a large bowl, sprinkle with sea salt, and drizzle with a little olive oil, tossing to coat. Serve at once. (This can be made in advance and stored well-covered in the refrigerator. Just before serving, reheat in the microwave.)

Braised eggplant with capers

SERVES 4

PREPARATION TIME
25 minutes (note sauce is made day in advance)

COOKING TIME
30 minutes

INGREDIENTS
1 can (14½ oz) diced tomatoes
olive oil
2 tbsp finely chopped garlic
2 small white onions, finely diced
3 celery ribs, finely diced
1 tbsp chopped fresh thyme
⅓ cup red wine vinegar
3 tbsp tomato paste
1½ tbsp fructose
1 cup green olives, pitted
1 (4 oz) jar capers, drained, rinsed, and chopped coarsely
1 cup flat-leaf parsley, chopped
4 medium or 8 small eggplant, cut into 1-in dice

ACCEPTABLE FOR
  RAPID WEIGHT LOSS
and

  WEIGHT CONTROL

This tomato-based sauce is prepared a day in advance and refrigerated to let the bold flavors develop—all the better to contrast with the smoky eggplant.

1 Drain the tomatoes in a sieve set over a bowl, pushing down gently to release the juice. Reserve the tomato pulp.

2 Heat 1 tablespoon olive oil in a large, heavy-bottomed saucepan over medium-high heat. Stir in the garlic, onions, celery, and thyme. Cook, covered, 3 to 5 minutes, until softened but not browned.

3 Pour in the strained tomato juice, and cook uncovered over medium-high heat until liquid is reduced in volume by ⅔. Stir in the red wine vinegar, reserved tomato pulp, tomato paste, and fructose to balance the tomato's acidity. Reduce the heat to low and add the olives, capers, and parsley. Check the seasonings and add salt to taste. Remove from the heat. Cool slightly, then transfer to a covered container and refrigerate overnight.

4 Preheat the oven to 500°F. Arrange the eggplant on a large baking sheet. Sprinkle with salt and drizzle with olive oil. Roast the eggplant in the oven, stirring once or twice, about 16 minutes or until tender and slightly browned. Let cool.

5 In a large bowl, mix the eggplant with the tomato sauce. Just before serving, drizzle with a little olive oil.

Red cabbage in red wine with walnuts and raisins

SERVES 4

PREPARATION TIME
30 minutes

COOKING TIME
25 minutes

INGREDIENTS

olive oil

1 onion, finely chopped

1 red cabbage, quartered, cored, and finely shredded

⅓ cup red wine vinegar plus a little extra to finish

2 cups dry red wine

1 (3-in) cinnamon stick

3½ oz fructose

⅓ cup (3½ oz) seedless golden raisins

½ cup toasted walnuts, chopped

3 tbsp herbes de Provence

2 tbsp shredded fresh sage leaves

good-quality walnut oil

ACCEPTABLE FOR

WEIGHT CONTROL

The appeal of this tasty salad is enhanced by lightly cooked red cabbage. It can also be made a day in advance with only a couple of finishing touches needed before serving.

1 Heat 1 tablespoon olive oil in a large, heavy-bottomed saucepan or Dutch oven over medium heat. Add the onion and cook 3 to 5 minutes, until just softened but not browned. Stir in the cabbage (or, using pot holders, simply invert the pan with the lid on, then turn right side up to mix). Add salt to taste, red wine vinegar, red wine, and the cinnamon stick. Reduce heat to low and cook, covered, until just tender, about 20 minutes.

2 Add 2 tablespoons of the herbes de Provence, and cook, uncovered, stirring until the liquid has evaporated slightly. Taste for seasoning, then add the fructose and raisins. When the cabbage is tender, pour into a serving bowl and let cool completely. (The salad can be made up to this point and stored in the refrigerator, covered, up to 24 hours.)

3 Remove the cinnamon stick and stir in the walnuts, sage, remaining 1 teaspoon herbes de Provence, and a splash of red wine vinegar.

4 Just before serving, drizzle a little walnut oil over the top.

Rice-stuffed onions

SERVES 4

PREPARATION TIME
25 minutes

COOKING TIME
50 minutes

INGREDIENTS

4 large red onions, peeled but left whole

2 tsp olive oil

1 tbsp balsamic vinegar

3 cups chicken stock

6 tbsp (3 oz) unsalted butter

¾ cup brown rice

½ white onion, chopped

1 cup freshly grated Parmesan cheese

½ bunch of fresh thyme, chopped (about 1 tbsp)

½ bunch of fresh rosemary, chopped (about 1 tbsp)

½ bunch of fresh chives, chopped (about 1 tbsp)

½ bunch of fresh tarragon, chopped (about 1 tbsp)

2 tbsp (¾ oz) toasted pine nuts

2 tbsp (¾ oz) dried cranberries

ACCEPTABLE FOR

WEIGHT CONTROL

Roasting onions before stuffing them brings out their sweetness, which is perfectly offset by this cheesy herb-infused rice stuffing. The pine nuts add crunchiness to the texture of the dish, while the cranberries impart their distinctive tartness.

1 Preheat the oven to 350°F. Place the whole onions in a baking dish and drizzle with the olive oil and balsamic vinegar. Cover with foil and bake 30 minutes. Remove from the oven and let cool slightly.

2 Meanwhile, prepare the rice. Heat the chicken stock in a saucepan and keep warm. Melt the butter in a large, heavy-bottomed saucepan over medium heat. Add the onions and cook, stirring, until softened but not browned. Add the rice. Cook, stirring, until the rice is translucent and coated with butter, about 2 minutes. Gradually add the hot stock about ½ cup at a time, stirring continuously, until the rice is swollen and tender. Stir in the Parmesan, chopped herbs, pine nuts, and cranberries. Add salt to taste. Keep warm.

3 Using a sharp knife, slice the tops off the cooked onions and reserve. Scoop out the center of each onion to leave a ½-inch shell. Fill the onion cavities with the rice mixture, then top each one with the reserved tops. Return onions to the baking dish and bake until heated through, about 15 minutes. Serve on warmed plates.

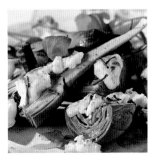

SERVES 4

PREPARATION TIME
35 minutes

COOKING TIME
20 minutes

INGREDIENTS
2 lemons, halved

8 globe artichokes

5-7 oz soft goat cheese

olive oil

2 tbsp chopped fresh chives

8 oz tender salad greens
such as arugula, endive, or
frisée, shredded

ACCEPTABLE FOR

RAPID WEIGHT LOSS
and

WEIGHT CONTROL

Artichoke hearts
with goat cheese

You could use ready-cooked artichoke hearts for this dish, but fresh ones are much better, if they are available. And there is no need to be intimidated by preparing them—it is a quick and simple process, and well worth the effort.

1 Fill a medium bowl with cold water and add the juice of 1 lemon. Cut off and discard all but ¼-inch of each artichoke stem. Rub the cut ends with the remaining lemon halves. One by one, carefully pull back the artichoke leaves until they break off naturally. Continue removing leaves until you reach the tender, pale green "heart." Using a serrated knife, cut off the top ¼-inch of the artichokes.

2 Cut the artichokes in half from tip to stem. With a spoon, scrape out the fuzzy choke. Rub the cut parts with lemon as you work. Turn the halves over, and with a small, sharp knife, trim away any tough, dark green outer parts. Place the artichoke halves in the bowl of water.

3 Bring a large, deep pot of salted water to a boil over high heat. Add the lemon halves and the trimmed artichoke halves. Cover and reduce heat to low. Cook until artichokes are just tender when pierced with the tip of a sharp knife, 15 to 20 minutes. Immediately drain in a colander.

4 Position the oven rack 6-inches above the boiler and preheat. In a bowl, mash the cheese with the chives. Add salt and freshly ground black pepper to taste.

5 Place the artichokes in an oiled baking dish and top with crumbled cheese. Broil, checking frequently, until the cheese is softened and the artichokes are lightly browned at the edges, about 5 to 7 minutes.

6 Serve on individual plates on a bed of salad greens.

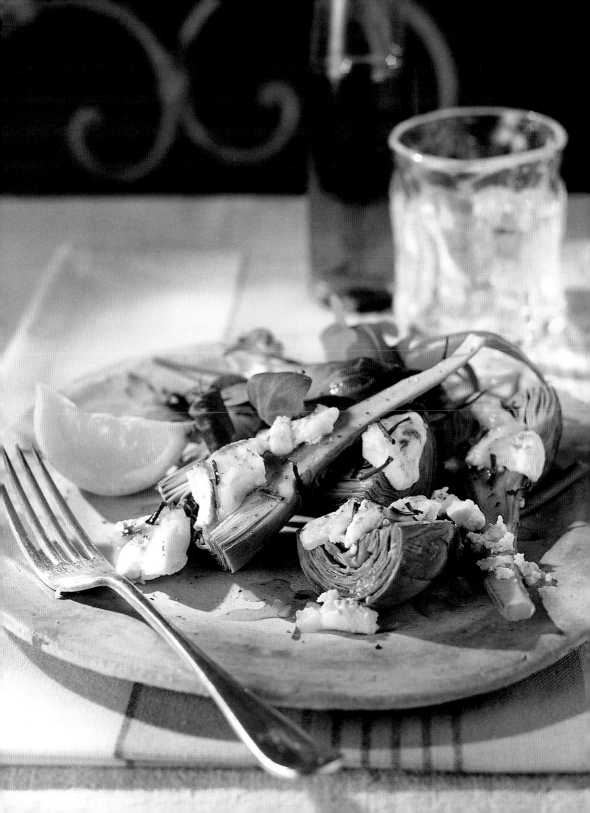

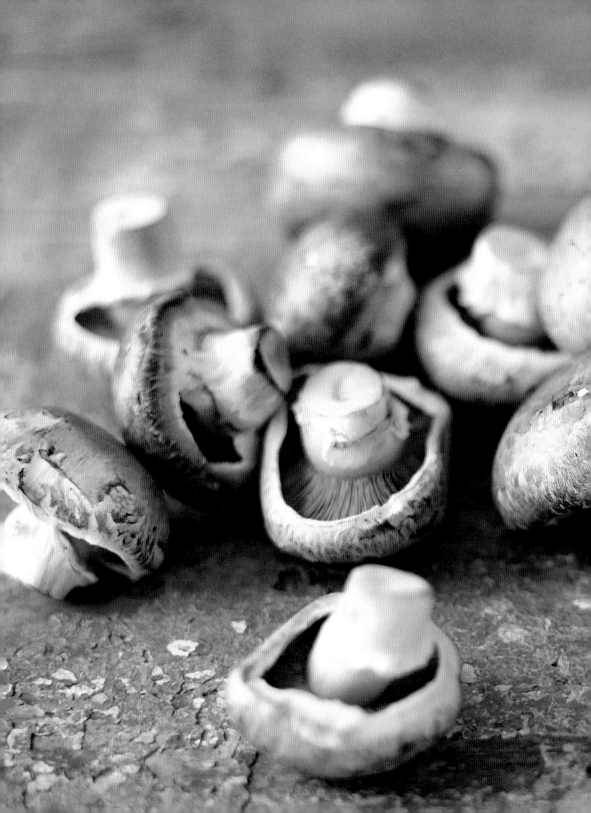

Main dishes

The following dishes range from quick-and-easy recipes to hearty French classics. Rich and flavorful, each recipe is compatible with the diet. The protein-based recipes are acceptable for both programs, but the pasta and rice dishes (*see pp192–95*) have a moderate fat content and are therefore suitable for the Weight Control Plan only.

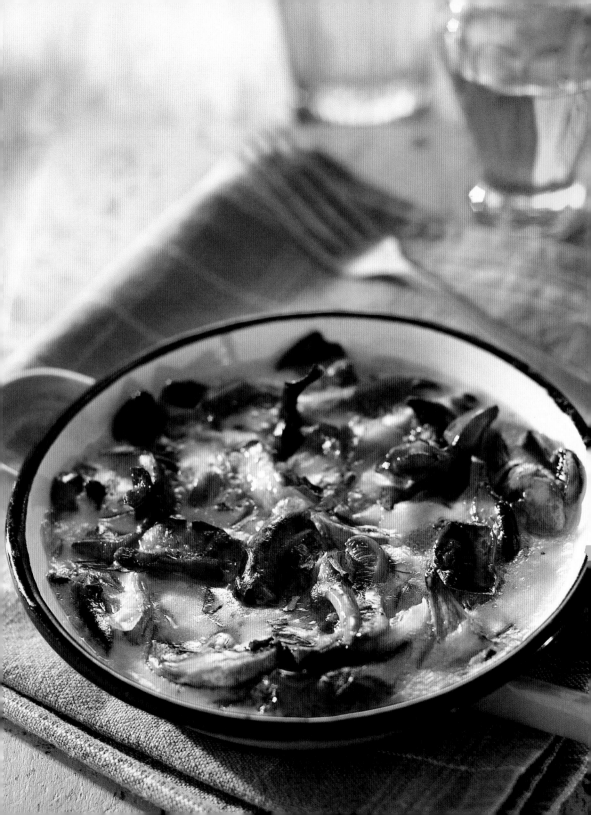

Wild mushroom custards

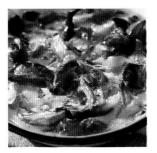

SERVES 4

PREPARATION TIME
20 minutes

COOKING TIME
30 minutes

INGREDIENTS
1½ lb wild mushrooms (such as shiitake, chanterelle, or oyster), trimmed and sliced

½ medium white onion, finely chopped

olive oil

salt

1 tbsp chopped fresh basil

1 tbsp chopped fresh chives

1 tbsp chopped fresh tarragon

4 oz large eggs

½ cup crème fraîche

butter for greasing

ACCEPTABLE FOR
  RAPID WEIGHT LOSS
and

  WEIGHT CONTROL

There is no longer any need to trek through the woods in search of wild mushrooms. Varieties ranging from the chewy, delicate chanterelle to the more robust oyster mushroom are often available at farmers' markets and upscale grocers.

1 Lightly grease 4 (8 ounce) glass or ceramic ramekins with butter. Preheat the oven to 300°F.

2 Heat 1½ tablespoons olive oil in a large skillet over medium–high heat. Add the mushrooms and onions, then season with salt. Cook, stirring frequently, until the onion is softened but not browned, about 5 minutes.

3 Drain the mushroom and onion mixture in a sieve. Transfer mixture to a bowl and set aside to cool. When it has cooled to room temperature, stir in the basil, chives, and tarragon.

4 In a medium bowl, combine the eggs, crème fraîche, and a pinch of salt. Stir in the mushroom mixture.

5 Divide the mixture between the 4 ramekins, then place them in a roasting pan filled with enough water to reach halfway up the sides of the ramekins. Carefully place in the oven and bake for 20 to 25 minutes, until the tops are slightly browned and the centers show no evidence of uncooked eggs. Serve hot.

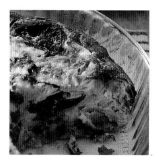

Montignac Gruyère quiche

Slow-cooking tomatoes develop a sweet, intense flavor that pairs well with the herbs and garlic.

SERVES 4

PREPARATION TIME
25 minutes

COOKING TIME
2 hours 45 minutes

INGREDIENTS
10 ripe tomatoes, halved and seeded

olive oil

1 tsp minced fresh garlic

1 tsp herbes de Provence

1 white onion, finely chopped

½ lb thick-sliced bacon cut crosswise into ¼-in pieces or pancetta cut into ½-in cubes

8 large eggs

2 cups crème fraîche or heavy (whipping) cream

2 tbsp canned tomato purée or sauce

1 tbsp chopped fresh chives

1 cup shredded Gruyère cheese

ACCEPTABLE FOR
RAPID WEIGHT LOSS
and

WEIGHT CONTROL

1 Lightly grease a 10-inch round baking dish. Preheat the oven to 300°F.

2 To make the provençal tomatoes, arrange the tomato halves cut-side up on a baking sheet. Drizzle with olive oil, then sprinkle with the garlic, herbes de Provence, and salt. Bake 1½ to 2 hours. Set aside to cool. Do not turn off the oven.

3 Heat 1 tablespoon of olive oil in a large skillet over medium heat. Add the onion and cook 3 to 5 minutes, until softened but not browned. Transfer to a sieve to drain.

4 Add the bacon to the skillet and cook over high heat 5 to 7 minutes, until nicely browned. Drain on paper towels.

5 Break the eggs into a large bowl. Whisk in the crème fraîche and tomato purée. Stir in the chives, bacon, and onion.

6 Arrange the slow-roasted tomatoes in the baking dish and scatter the cheese over the top. Pour in the egg mixture. (Tomatoes will float to the top.) Bake 30 to 40 minutes, until the top is golden brown and the custard shows no evidence of uncooked egg. Let cool slightly before cutting into pie-shaped wedges. This quiche is also delicious served cold.

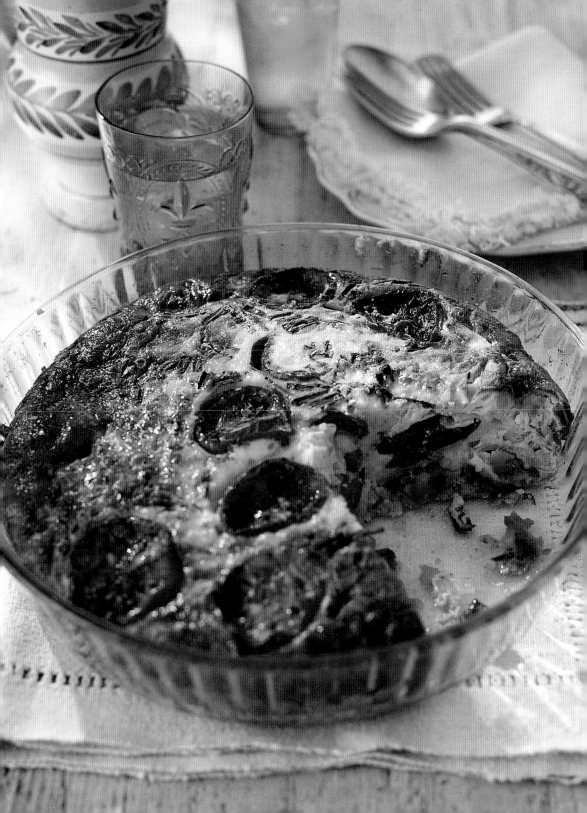

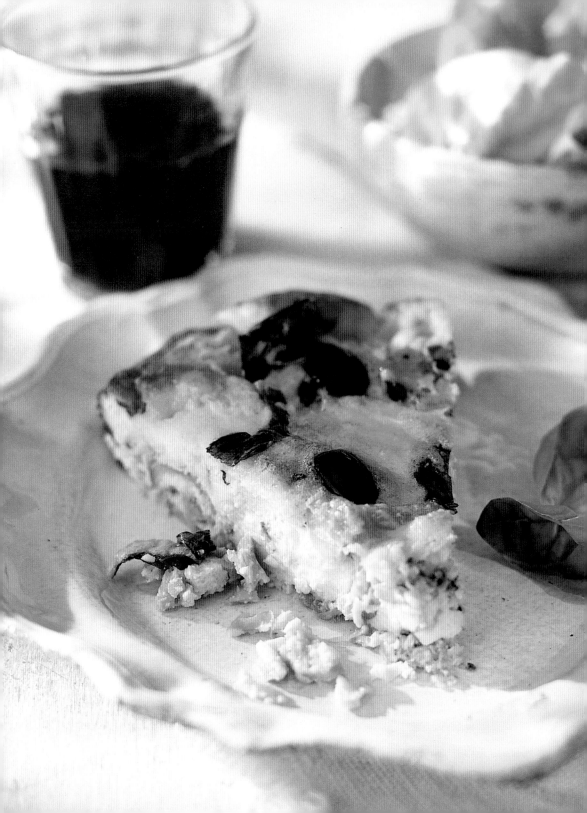

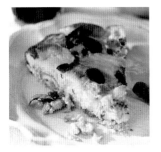

Salmon and blue cheese quiche

SERVES 4

PREPARATION TIME
20 minutes

COOKING TIME
40 minutes

INGREDIENTS
1 white onion, chopped

olive oil

⅔ cup freshly grated Parmesan cheese

2 tbsp chopped fresh basil

8 large eggs, beaten

2 cups crème fraîche or heavy (whipping) cream

10 black olives, pitted and halved

10½ oz thinly sliced smoked salmon, cut into bite-size pieces

1 cup Roquefort or blue cheese, diced or crumbled

ACCEPTABLE FOR
RAPID WEIGHT LOSS
and

WEIGHT CONTROL

Smoked salmon and crème fraîche make a classic combination reminiscent of smoked salmon and cream cheese. When the sharp flavors of olives and Roquefort cheese are introduced to the mix, you have a filling, sense-satisfying quiche.

1 Lightly grease a 10-inch round baking dish with butter. Preheat the oven to 300°F.

2 Heat 1 tablespoon olive oil in a large skillet over medium heat. Add the onion and cook 3 to 5 minutes, until softened but not browned. Scrape the onion mixture into a large bowl to cool before stirring in the Parmesan and basil.

3 In a separate bowl, beat together the eggs and crème fraîche until well blended. Pour into the onion mixture; add the olives and mix well. Gently stir in the salmon.

4 Pour the egg mixture into the buttered dish. Sprinkle the Roquefort over the mixture—the cheese should float to the top. Bake 30 to 40 minutes, or until the top is golden brown and the custard shows no evidence of uncooked egg. Cool to room temperature before serving.

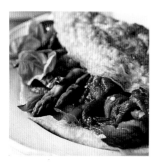

SERVES 4

PREPARATION TIME
30 minutes

COOKING TIME
45 minutes

INGREDIENTS
2 large red bell peppers
olive oil
½ lb asparagus, woody ends
trimmed, cut into 2-in lengths
½ white onion, chopped
12 large eggs
2 tbsp chopped fresh basil
plus extra leaves for garnish
⅓ cup heavy (whipping)
cream
½ cup freshly grated
Parmesan cheese

ACCEPTABLE FOR
 RAPID WEIGHT LOSS
and

 WEIGHT CONTROL

Omelette with red peppers and asparagus

This satisfying egg dish can be made in two ways: as a classic omelette stuffed with peppers, basil, and asparagus; or like a frittata, with the egg and vegetables combined and baked in the oven at 300°F for 20 to 30 minutes.

1 Preheat the oven to 500°F. Cut the peppers in half lengthwise and remove the stems and seeds. Place them cut-side down on a baking sheet. Roast 20 minutes, or until the skins are charred. Remove and set aside. When cool enough to handle, rub off the skins and cut into ½-inch strips.

2 Bring a pot of salted water to a boil over high heat. Add asparagus and cook until bright green and crisp-tender, 2 to 3 minutes. Drain quickly, then plunge into ice water to refresh. Drain again and set aside.

3 Heat 2 tablespoons olive oil in a medium skillet over medium heat. Add the onion and cook, stirring occasionally, until softened but not browned, 3 to 5 minutes. Set aside.

4 In a large bowl, whisk eggs with cream to blend. Stir in the basil, Parmesan, and a pinch of salt.

5 To make one large omelette: In a deep, 12-inch skillet, heat 1½ tablespoons olive oil over medium heat. Pour in the egg mixture and let sit 1 minute. Using a heatproof rubber spatula, carefully lift the edges away from the sides of the pan, letting the uncooked eggs flow to the bottom. Cook until the omelette is almost set but still moist on top, 12 to 15 minutes. Scatter the peppers, asparagus, and onion over one half, fold the omelette over the top, and slide out of the pan onto a warmed serving plate. Cut into 4 pieces, garnish with the extra basil, and serve.

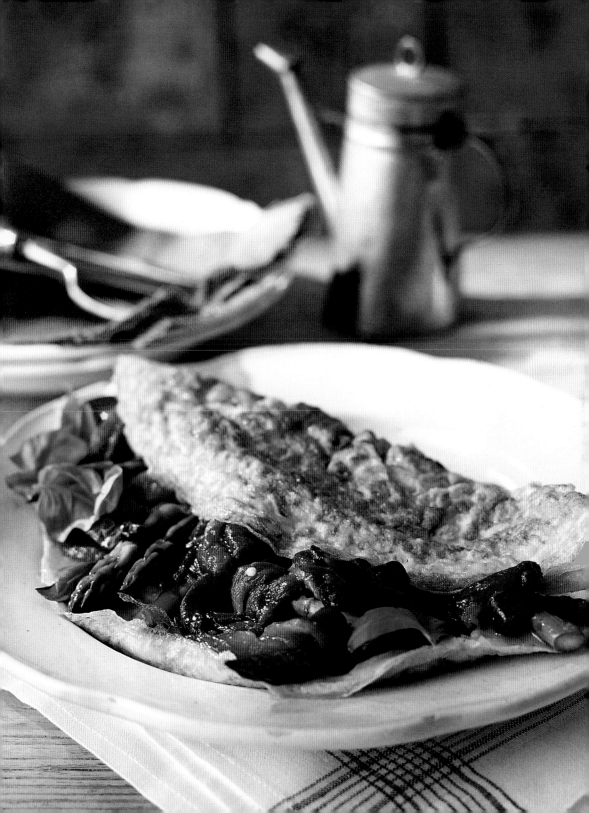

Pasta with tuna and artichokes

SERVES 4

PREPARATION TIME
15 minutes

COOKING TIME
8 minutes

INGREDIENTS

grated zest and juice of
2 lemons

⅓ cup olive oil

10 lb whole wheat pasta,
such as spaghetti

salt

2 (6 oz) cans tuna, drained

1 (15 oz) can artichoke
hearts, drained and halved

¼ cup julienne-cut, oil packed
sun-dried tomatoes

15 kalamata olives, pitted
(⅓ cup)

2 tablespoons capers, rinsed

½ cup flat-leaf parsley,
chopped

ACCEPTABLE FOR

WEIGHT CONTROL

The key to this dish is cooking the pasta just before serving—be sure to have all the other elements prepared and ready to go. Once the pasta is cooked, you need to move quickly. The lemon mixture is added first so the hot pasta absorbs its flavor and heavenly aroma.

1 In a small bowl, combine the lemon zest and juice, olive oil, and salt.

2 Bring a large pot of salted water to a boil over high heat. Add the pasta and cook 12 to 15 minutes, until *al dente*—do not overcook. Drain in a colander, reserving ½ cup of the cooking water. Quickly return the pasta to the pot with the reserved cooking water, and season with salt and freshly ground black pepper.

3 Add the lemon-oil mixture, tossing gently to coat. Stir in the tuna, artichokes, sun-dried tomatoes, olives, capers, and parsley. Serve at once in a large, shallow, warmed bowl.

Tricolor rice with balsamic onions

SERVES 4

PREPARATION TIME
10 minutes

COOKING TIME
30 minutes

INGREDIENTS

1¼ cups long-grain brown rice

1¼ cups Basmati rice

⅔ cup wild rice

olive oil

3 white onions, finely chopped

2 cups balsamic vinegar

ACCEPTABLE FOR

WEIGHT CONTROL

This is an appetizing and slightly different way to serve rice, with its sticky, caramelized onions and blending of textures and flavors in the rice itself. It is just as good when it is reheated as it is served fresh from the pan the first time around.

1   Put each rice into its own heavy-bottomed saucepan. Gently pour in enough cold water to cover by 2-inches. Cover each pot and bring to a boil; then continue cooking at a steady but not too vigorous boil for 16 to 20 minutes, or until rice is tender. Combine all the rice in a fine sieve or colander and drain off any liquid. Cool with cold running water and drain again.

2   Heat a large frying pan or wok over high heat. Add 1 tablespoon oil. Add the onions and fry, stirring and tossing, 5 to 7, minutes or until golden. Pour in the balsamic vinegar and cook, stirring frequently, until the onion is dark and sticky and most of the liquid has evaporated, 10 to 12 minutes.

3   Stir the rice into the onion mixture. Season with salt to taste. Serve at once, or cover and refrigerate. Reheat in a microwave or wok.

Linguini with ratatouille

SERVES 4

PREPARATION TIME
35 minutes

COOKING TIME
45 minutes

INGREDIENTS
olive oil

1 onion, finely chopped

3 garlic cloves, finely chopped

1 tbsp chopped fresh thyme

4 red bell peppers, cut into ½-in dice

4 yellow bell peppers, cut into ½-in dice

1 large eggplant, cut into ½-in dice

2 zucchini, cut into ½-in dice

1 can (14½ oz) tomato pureé

1 fresh bay leaf

¾ cup (10½ oz) whole wheat linguini

dash of sherry vinegar

dash of red wine vinegar

2 tbsp fresh flat-leaf parsley, chopped

1 cup cherry tomatoes, halved and drained in a colander

1 cup grated Parmesan cheese

ACCEPTABLE FOR

WEIGHT CONTROL

This classic French vegetable stew makes a memorable complement to nutty whole wheat pasta. Once all the ingredients have been chopped, the dish goes together quite nicely.

1 To make the ratatouille, heat 2 tablespoons olive oil in a heavy-bottomed saucepan over medium heat. When the oil is hot, add the onion, garlic, and thyme. Cook, stirring, 3 minutes. Stir in the peppers. Cook, covered, 5 minutes to soften. Stir in the eggplant and zucchini. Add salt to taste. Stir in the tomato pureé and bay leaf. Reduce heat to low and simmer, uncovered, 30 minutes.

2 Bring a large pot of salted water to a boil over high heat. Add the linguine and cook 10 to 12 minutes, until *al dente*. Drain in a colander, reserving ½ cup of the cooking water.

3 Return pasta to the pot with the reserved cooking water, and, while it is still hot, add 1½ tablespoons olive oil. Stir in the sherry vinegar and red wine vinegar. Add salt to taste.

4 Quickly stir the parsley and cherry tomatoes into the ratatouille. Discard the bay leaf.

5 To serve, divide pasta among 4 warmed shallow bowls. Top each with ratatouille and drizzle with a teaspoon of olive oil. Pass Parmesan cheese at the table.

Penne with capers and olives

SERVES 4

PREPARATION TIME
15 minutes

COOKING TIME
6–8 minutes

INGREDIENTS

juice of 2 lemons

salt

½ cup olive oil

¾ cup (10½ oz) whole wheat penne

¼ cup julienne-cut, oil packed sun-dried tomatoes

5 cloves garlic, finely chopped

20 kalamata olives, pitted (about ½ cup)

20 green olives, pitted (about ½ cup)

3–4 tbsp capers, rinsed and drained

½ cup flat-leaf parsley, chopped

pinch of hot red pepper flakes (optional)

ACCEPTABLE FOR

WEIGHT CONTROL

Another dish with a strong provençal influence, this fresh-tasting pasta is packed with clean, strong flavors that do not overwhelm. The red pepper flakes add a little heat, but can be omitted if you prefer a milder flavor.

1 In a bowl, combine the lemon juice, a pinch of salt, and olive oil.

2 Bring a large pot of salted water to a boil over high heat. Add the penne and cook about 12 minutes, until *al dente*. Drain in a colander, reserving about ½ cup of the cooking water.

3 Return the penne to the pot with the reserved cooking water, and season with salt and freshly ground black pepper. Stir in the lemon-oil mixture, the sun-dried tomatoes, garlic, olives, capers, parsley, and pepper flakes. Toss to coat. Divide pasta among 4 warmed pasta bowls and serve at once.

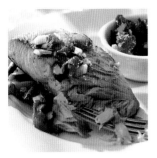

Salmon provençale

A little chopping, a little whisking, a few minutes in the oven, and this dish is ready to go. The technique may be simple, but this beautiful presentation is only surpassed by its sophisticated flavors.

SERVES 4

PREPARATION TIME
20 minutes

COOKING TIME
12 minutes

INGREDIENTS
3 large tomatoes
3 shallots, coarsely chopped
1 tbsp coarsely chopped fresh chervil
1 tbsp coarsely chopped fresh basil
1 tbsp coarsely chopped fresh tarragon
1 tbsp coarsely chopped fresh chives
juice of ½ lemon
1½ tbsp balsamic vinegar
salt
2 tbsp olive oil, plus extra for drizzling
4 salmon fillets, about 5-6 oz each

ACCEPTABLE FOR
RAPID WEIGHT LOSS
and

WEIGHT CONTROL

1 Preheat the oven to 400°F.

2 Blanch the tomatoes by plunging them into a pot of boiling salted water for 15 to 30 seconds, then plunging into ice water for 1 minute. Drain the tomatoes and peel off and discard the skin. Cut the tomatoes into quarters, remove the core (including seeds), and dice the flesh.

3 In a large bowl, combine the tomato, shallots, chervil, basil, tarragon, and chives.

4 In a small bowl, whisk together the lemon juice, balsamic vinegar, and salt to taste. Whisk in the 2 tablespoons olive oil until well blended. Add to the tomato mixture, tossing gently to coat.

5 Arrange salmon on an oiled baking sheet without crowding. Drizzle with olive oil and season lightly with salt. Bake until salmon is barely cooked through and lightly browned at the edges, 10 to 12 minutes.

6 To serve, drain the salmon on paper towels to absorb any excess oil, then place a fillet on each of 4 warmed dinner plates. Spoon 1 to 2 tablespoons of the tomato mixture over each. Serve at once.

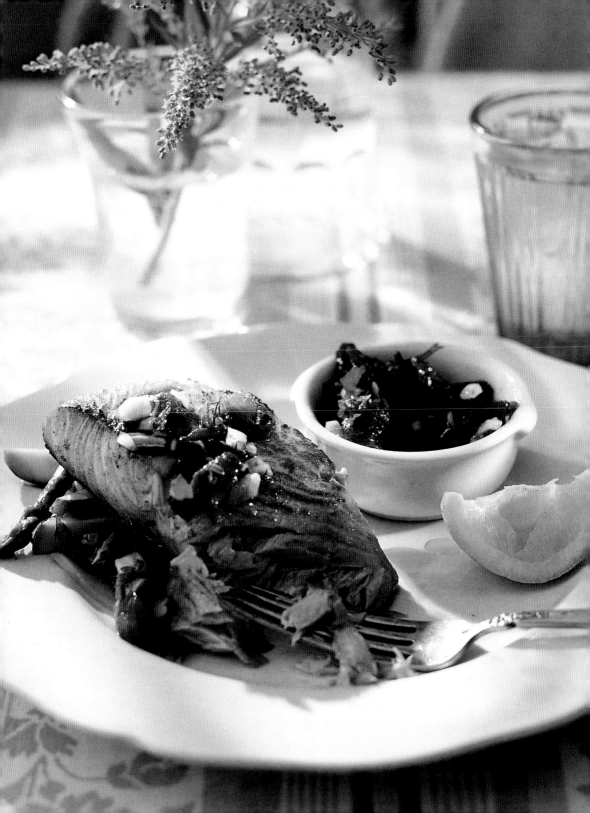

Cod on a bed of lentils

SERVES 4

PREPARATION TIME
25 minutes

COOKING TIME
40 minutes

INGREDIENTS
½ cup green lentils,
preferably Lentilles du Puy
(small french lentils), cooked
(see p. 176)

12 ripe cherry tomatoes

8 thin slices pancetta

olive oil

4 cod fillets, skin on,
(4-6 oz each)

juice of ½ lemon

2½ cups (4 oz) fresh baby
spinach leaves

pinch of freshly grated
nutmeg

FRESH TOMATO SAUCE
2 tsp olive oil

1 onion, chopped

3 celery ribs, chopped

1 lb ripe tomatoes, seeded
and chopped

2 tbsp each chopped fresh
basil and tarragon

1 can (14½ oz) diced
tomatoes, drained

juice of 1 lemon

¼ cup white wine vinegar

ACCEPTABLE FOR
RAPID WEIGHT LOSS
and

WEIGHT CONTROL

This is a dish of layered flavors, each one complementing the others. If cod is unavailable, choose another delicate white fish fillet, such as snapper or halibut. Baking the pancetta between two baking sheets helps keep it flat, rather than curling during cooking.

1 To make the tomato sauce: In a large, heavy-bottomed saucepan, heat the onion and celery and cook, stirring occasionally, until softened but not browned, 3 to 5 minutes. Stir in the tomatoes, basil, and tarragon. Cook, stirring occasionally, 5 minutes. Add the canned tomatoes, lemon juice, and white wine vinegar. Reduce heat to low and cook 20 minutes, or until a thick sauce has formed. Keep warm.

2 Preheat the oven to 475°F. Place the cherry tomatoes on a baking sheet. Sprinkle with salt and drizzle with olive oil. Lay the pancetta on another baking sheet, then place a same-sized sheet on top. Roast the cherry tomatoes in the oven 5 to 7 minutes, or just until the skins start to split. Remove from the oven and put in the double tray of pancetta. Bake 6 minutes, until the pancetta is crispy. Reduce oven temperature to 400°F.

3 Arrange cod on an oiled baking sheet without crowding. Drizzle with olive oil and season with salt. Bake until cod is just cooked through, 10 to 12 minutes.

4 Heat 1 tablespoon olive oil in a heavy-bottomed saucepan over medium-high heat. Add lentils and cook, stirring, until heated through, 2 to 3 minutes. Stir in the spinach, lemon juice, and nutmeg, and cook just until the spinach has wilted, 1 to 2 minutes.

5 Divide the lentil-spinach mixture among 4 warmed plates. Top each with a cod fillet. Crisscross the pancetta slices over the cod. Drizzle fresh tomato sauce around the fish and serve at once.

Grilled sea bass with tapenade

SERVES 4

PREPARATION TIME
30 minutes, plus 2 hours
for marinating

COOKING TIME
10 minutes

INGREDIENTS
4 sea bass steaks, skin on,
about 4-6 oz each
1 tbsp each chopped fresh
chervil, basil, and tarragon

FOR THE MARINADE
1 tsp ground coriander
3 garlic cloves, chopped
juice of 1 lemon
¼ cup olive oil

FOR THE TAPENADE
1½ cups kalamata olives,
pitted
2 tbsp drained capers
4 flat anchovy filets, drained
3 garlic cloves
2 tbsp chopped fresh parsley
juice of ½ lemon
¼ cup olive oil

ACCEPTABLE FOR
RAPID WEIGHT LOSS
and

WEIGHT CONTROL

For this recipe, the sea bass can be cooked on an indoor or outdoor grill, under a broiler, or in a hot oven. Either way, the combination of marinade and tapenade keeps the fish moist.

1 In a glass or ceramic dish, mix together the lemon juice, garlic, coriander, and olive oil. Add fish steaks, turning to coat. Marinate covered in the refrigerator up to 2 hours.

2 To prepare the tapenade: In a food processor, combine the olives, capers, anchovies, garlic, parsley, lemon juice, and olive oil. Process, pulsing the machine on and off, until a coarse paste forms. Transfer to a small bowl and refrigerate until needed.

3 Preheat the oven to 400°F. Remove fish from marinade and pat dry. Arrange sea bass steaks on an oiled baking sheet without crowding. Season lightly with salt. Bake until the fish is just cooked through, about 10 minutes.

4 Brush each piece of fish with 1 teaspoon of tapenade.

5 To serve, place a fish steak on each of 4 warmed serving plates and top with a spoonful of tapenade. Scatter herbs over the top and serve at once.

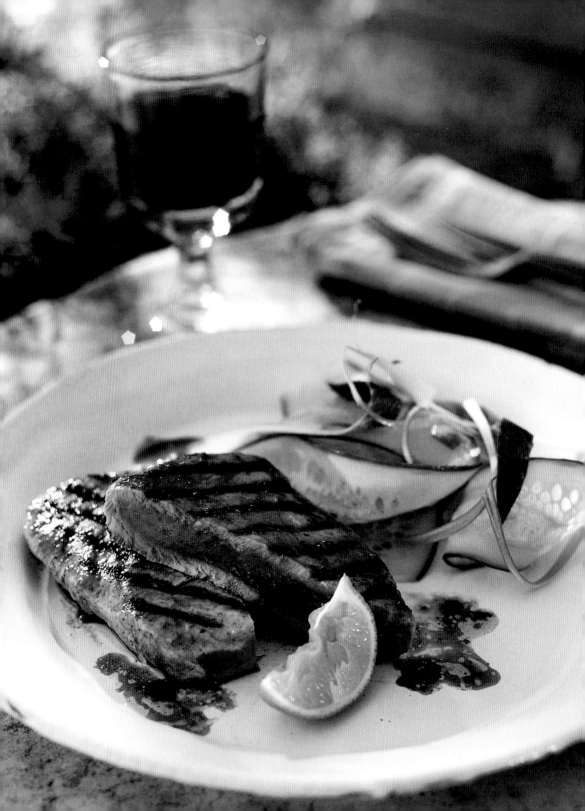

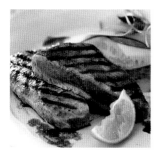

Grilled tuna with Mediterranean marinade

Tuna is a meaty fish, similar in texture to steak. After soaking up a simple marinade of lemon and olive oil, the tuna steaks are coated with a spicy rub before being broiled.

SERVES 4

PREPARATION TIME
10 minutes, plus 2 hours for marinating

COOKING TIME
8 minutes

INGREDIENTS
4 red tuna steaks, (6-8 oz and about 1½ in thick)
juice of 1½ lemons
3 tbsp olive oil

MEDITERRANEAN RUB
3 garlic cloves, crushed through a press
2 tsp ground cumin
2 tsp grated fresh ginger
¼ tsp saffron threads or ground coriander
salt and pepper

ACCEPTABLE FOR
RAPID WEIGHT LOSS
and

WEIGHT CONTROL

1 Place the fish in a glass or ceramic dish with the lemon juice and olive oil. Marinate, covered, in the refrigerator for a few hours.

2 To make the rub: In a small bowl, combine the garlic, cumin, ginger saffron, salt, and freshly ground black pepper to taste. Mix well to blend.

3 Position the top oven rack 4-inches from the heat source. Preheat the broiler. Coat both sides of each tuna steak with the rub. Arrange on an oiled broiler pan without crowding. Broil, turning once, until lightly browned on the outside and cooked to desired doneness inside, 6 to 8 minutes total for medium rare.

4 Transfer tuna steaks to 4 warmed dinner plates and serve at once.

Prawns à la pastis

SERVES 4

PREPARATION TIME
25 minutes

COOKING TIME
15 minutes

INGREDIENTS
1 tbsp fennel seed
2 fennel bulbs, including greenery
olive oil
16 large prawns (about 1 lb), peeled and deveined
juice of ½ lemon
⅓ cup pastis or Pernod
2 tbsp (1 oz) cold unsalted butter, cut into ½-in cubes

ACCEPTABLE FOR
RAPID WEIGHT LOSS
and
WEIGHT CONTROL

Pastis, a licorice-flavored apéritif, is quite popular in the south of France. Its flavor is mimicked by the fennel, and intensified further by using freshly ground seeds, instead of store-bought ground fennel.

1 Roast fennel seeds in a dry skillet over medium heat, stirring, 1 minute or until fragrant. Remove from heat and let cool slightly. Grind to a fine powder using a mortar and pestle or a clean electric spice mill.

2 Trim the fennel bulbs, reserving any fronds for use later. Chop the bulbs finely.

3 Heat olive oil in a large skillet over medium-high heat. Season prawns with salt, and dust lightly with the ground roasted fennel seed. Cook, stirring and tossing, until prawns just turn pink and begin to curl, 3 to 4 minutes. Transfer to a plate and set aside.

4 Add the chopped fennel to the same pan and cook, stirring frequently, until softened, 3 to 5 minutes. Return the prawns to the pan and squeeze in the lemon juice. Standing back, slowly pour in the pastis (be careful as the alcohol may ignite). Cook, stirring, until the alcohol has evaporated.

5 Spoon the fennel and prawns into warmed shallow bowls. Add the cream to the pan and cook over medium-high heat, stirring frequently, until slightly thickened, about 2 minutes. Reduce heat to low. Gradually whisk in the cold butter one piece at a time, waiting until butter is melted and fully incorporated before the heat addition. Chop up to 2 teaspoons of the fennel fronds and add to the sauce. Pour over the prawns and serve at once.

Soup d'Atlantique

SERVES 4

PREPARATION TIME
30 minutes

COOKING TIME
25 minutes

INGREDIENTS
2 tsp olive oil

3 shallots, finely chopped

1 lb mussels, scrubbed and beards removed

⅔ cup dry white wine

2 cups good-quality fish stock

2 cups good-quality herb or white vegetable stock (see method)

1 star anise

3½ cups heavy (whipping) cream

2 tbsp chopped fresh dill

½ lb very fresh, firm white ocean fish, such as cod, halibut, or snapper, skinned, boned, and cut into ½-in pieces

¼ lb very fresh, tiny bay scallops or larger sea scallops, cut into ½-in pieces

ACCEPTABLE FOR

RAPID WEIGHT LOSS
and

WEIGHT CONTROL

In this satisfying soup, seafood lies like a treasure at the bottom of the bowls. It is easy enough to make your own herb stock, but if you choose not to, be sure to buy a good-quality stock that does not contain carrots.

1 Heat oil in a large, heavy-bottomed saucepan over medium heat. Add the shallots and cook, stirring, until softened, about 3 minutes. Increase heat to medium-high and add the mussels. When some of the mussels just begin to open, add the wine. Cook, covered, 4 to 5 minutes, or until the mussels are cooked. Transfer mussels to a bowl. Strain the mussel liquor and return to the pan.

2 Add the fish stock, herb stock, and star anise. Bring to a boil and cook over high heat until reduced by ½. Whisk in the cream and continue cooking until the stock begins to thicken, about 5 to 10 minutes. Add salt to taste if necessary. Reduce the heat to low and keep warm.

3 Divide the mussels and raw scallops and seafood between 4 shallow bowls. Return the soup to a boil. Ladle the hot soup into the bowls—this will poach the uncooked seafood. Sprinkle with dill and serve at once.

HERB STOCK Melt 1 tablespoon butter in a stockpot or saucepan over medium heat. Add 1 chopped leek, 2 chopped onions, ½ chopped celery rib, and 1 tablespoon chopped garlic. Cook for 5 to 6 minutes, stirring occasionally, until softened but not browned. Add 2 sprigs of fresh thyme, 1 parsley stalk, 1 teaspoon coriander seed, 1½ cups dry white wine, and a good pinch of salt. Cover with 2 cups cold water. Bring to a vigorous boil, then add 1 bunch each of fresh sage, basil, coriander, and dill. Add more salt if needed, to bring out the full flavor. Simmer over low heat for 30 minutes. Strain through a fine sieve, discarding the vegetables and herbs.

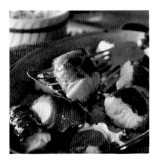

Fresh cod and prosciutto rolls

Wrapping the cod with prosciutto keeps the fish firmly in place as it cooks. The cod and prosciutto rolls contrast well with the robust flavor of spiced cabbage.

SERVES 4

PREPARATION TIME
25 minutes

COOKING TIME
15 minutes

INGREDIENTS

4 fresh cod or other firm, skinless white fish fillets, 6 oz each

salt and pepper

8 slices prosciutto or Parma ham

2 tbsp olive oil

1 lb savoy cabbage or kale, outer leaves and hard core removed, shredded

1 tsp cumin or fennel seed

1 tbsp chopped fresh thyme or parsley, plus extra for garnish

1 tbsp white wine vinegar

ACCEPTABLE FOR

RAPID WEIGHT LOSS
and

WEIGHT CONTROL

1 Cut each fillet in half. Season the fish with salt and pepper to taste (be careful, as the ham can be salty on its own). Wrap each piece of fish in the prosciutto slice, placing the fish along one short end of the ham and rolling up lengthwise.

2 Heat 1 tablespoon of the olive oil in a large skillet over medium-high heat. Add the fish and cook, turning once, until the ham is lightly browned and the fish is just cooked through, 6 to 8 minutes.

3 Meanwhile, place a metal steamer basket over simmering water in a large pot. Cook the cabbage, covered, for about 5 minutes, or just until wilted. Do not overcook.

4 In a small dry skillet, heat cumin seed over medium heat, stirring, until fragrant, about 1 minute.

5 In a warmed serving bowl, combine the cabbage, cumin seed, 1 tablespoon thyme, vinegar, and the remaining olive oil. Season with salt and freshly ground black pepper to taste. Toss gently to mix.

6 Make a bed of the cabbage on a warmed serving dish, arrange the cod rolls on top, and sprinkle with the extra thyme. Alternatively, serve cabbage on the side. Serve at once.

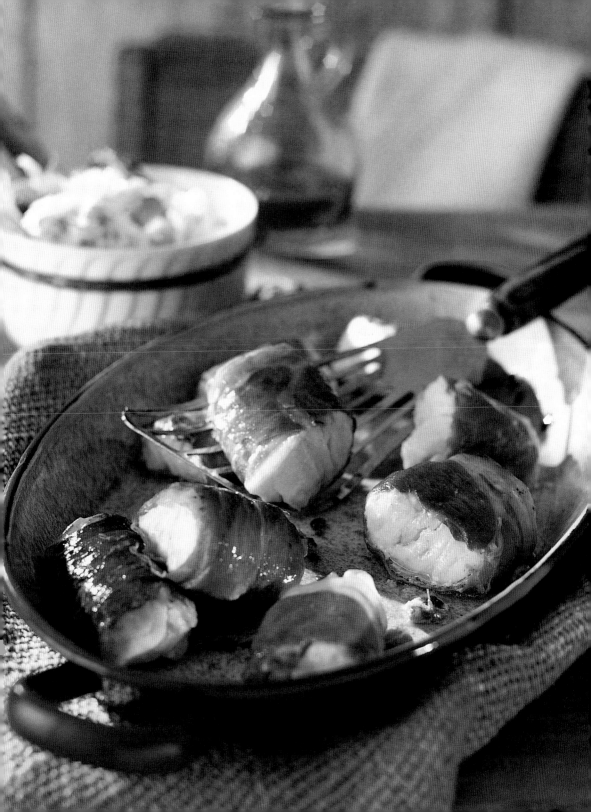

Chicken breasts in creamy garlic sauce

SERVES 4

PREPARATION TIME
10 minutes

COOKING TIME
50 minutes

INGREDIENTS

1 tbsp fresh tarragon, chopped, plus extra for garnish

1 tbsp fresh basil, chopped

1 tbsp of fresh chives, chopped

1 tbsp of fresh chervil, chopped

4 boneless chicken breasts with skin on, about 6 oz each

3 heads of garlic, cloves separated but unpeeled

2 cups milk

2 tbsp olive oil

2 cups heavy (whipping) cream

1½ tbsp paprika

ACCEPTABLE FOR
RAPID WEIGHT LOSS
and
WEIGHT CONTROL

Slow-roasting whole garlic cloves in milk not only softens them, but also rids them of any harsh flavor. The resulting sauce makes a creamy complement to the herb-packed grilled chicken.

1 Preheat the oven to 325°F. Rinse chicken with cold water and pat dry with paper towels. Mix together the tarragon, basil, chives, and chervil. Using a teaspoon or your fingers, push the herbs under the skins of the chicken breasts, trying not to tear the skin. Arrange chicken on a baking sheet and cover with plastic wrap. Refrigerate up to 4 hours.

2 Bring a saucepan of water to a boil over high heat. Add garlic cloves and cook until water returns to a boil, 1 to 2 minutes. Drain, discarding the water. Place garlic in a 2 quart ceramic baking dish. Drizzle with olive oil and cover with the milk. Cover with foil and bake 40 minutes, until the garlic is soft. Strain the garlic-infused milk into a small, heavy-bottomed saucepan. Squeeze the garlic cloves to extract the pulp, adding it to the milk. Bring to a simmer over low heat, whisking. Keep warm.

3 Heat a grill pan or griddle over medium-high heat. Season the chicken with freshly ground black pepper and salt to taste. Drizzle with remaining oil. Grill 4 to 5 minutes on each side, or until lightly browned on the outside and white throughout. Bring the garlic sauce back to a simmer and whisk in the cream and paprika. Bring to a boil over high heat, whisking frequently. Reduce heat to low and keep warm.

4 To serve, cut each chicken breast into crosswise diagonal slices. Pour some garlic sauce onto the bottom of each of 4 warmed plates. Fan out the chicken slices slightly, and set on top of the sauce. Garnish with tarragon. Serve at once.

Rustic duck à l'orange

SERVES 4

PREPARATION TIME
30 minutes

COOKING TIME
1½ hours

INGREDIENTS
2 Long Island ducklings,
about 5 lb each

2 tbsp chopped garlic

1 tbsp chopped fresh thyme,
plus extra for stuffing and
garnish

zest of 2 oranges, cut into
thin strips

1 orange, halved, plus a few
slices for garnish, if desired

olive oil

2 tbsp chopped fresh parsley

ORANGE SAUCE
1 tsp butter

6 shallots, finely chopped

grated zest of 2 oranges

2 tbsp fructose

¼ cup malt vinegar

3½ cups veal or chicken
stock

2 tbsp orange juice

juice of ½ lemon

salt

ACCEPTABLE FOR
RAPID WEIGHT LOSS
and

WEIGHT CONTROL

A rustic variation of a classic French dish need not be
daunting at all. In fact, it all comes together very easily. The
secret is to baste the duck frequently while it is cooking. This
keeps the dark meat moist and turns the skin a rich, crisp
golden brown.

1 Preheat the oven to 425°F. Rinse duck inside and out with cold water;
pat dry with paper towels. If desired, remove the wishbones with a
boning knife. Mix together the garlic, chopped thyme, and orange
zest. Using a teaspoon or your fingers, lift up the skin of each duck
and smear the garlic mixture over the breast meat and between the
legs. Season the outside of the duck with salt to taste, and rub some
of the garlic mixture over the outside of each one. Place an orange
half inside the cavity of each duck, together with a large sprig of
thyme. Truss with heavy cotton twine, closing the cavities and
bringing the legs together.

2 Place the ducks on their sides on a rack in a large roasting pan.
Drizzle each very lightly with olive oil and place in the oven. After
18 minutes, turn onto their other sides and roast for 18 minutes
longer. Lastly, turn onto their backs and roast 40 minutes, or until
done. Baste as they cook so the skin will turn a rich, golden brown.

3 Meanwhile, prepare the sauce. Melt the butter in a heavy-bottomed
saucepan over medium heat. Stir in the shallots and orange zest.
When mixture is bubbling-hot, sprinkle in the fructose and continue
to caramelize slightly. Stir in the malt vinegar, stock, and orange juice.
Bring the sauce to a simmer over medium-high heat until volume is
reduced by about about ⅓ and the sauce begins to thicken. Add the
lemon juice. Taste, adding salt as needed. Keep warm.

4 Carve the duck and arrange legs and breasts on 4 warmed plates. Lay
some orange slices over the top if desired. Sprinkle with parsley and
drizzle with sauce.

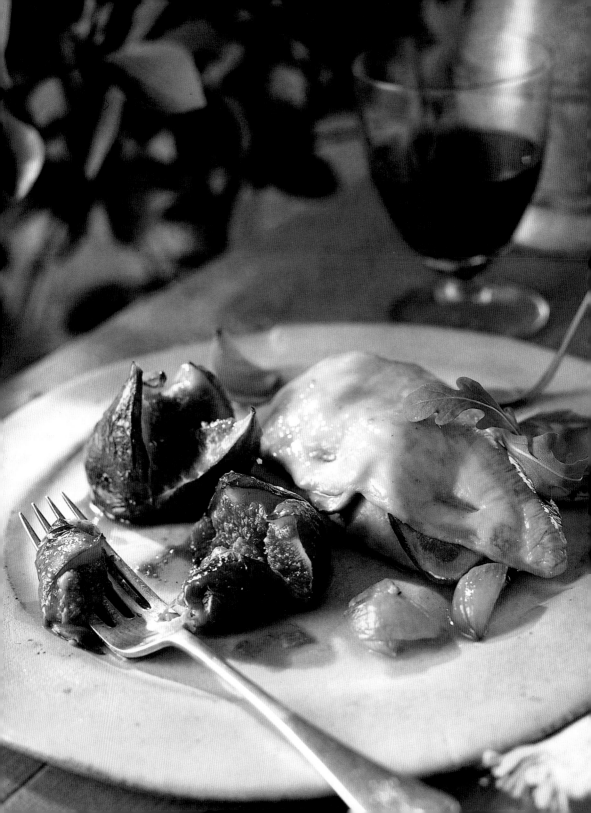

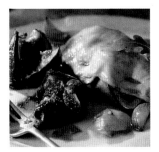

Chicken with figs

The juicy figs and fresh shallots complement each other, giving this chicken dish just the right balance of sweet and savory. In addition, wine keeps the chicken moist, while bringing out the subtle flavors of the other ingredients. .

SERVES 4

PREPARATION TIME
40 minutes

COOKING TIME
25 minutes

INGREDIENTS
4 boneless skinless chicken breast halves, about 6 oz each

8 fresh figs, sliced, plus 4 whole figs for garnish

olive oil

3 large shallots, sliced

⅓ cup dry white wine

⅓ stick (6 oz) cold unsalted butter, cut into ½-in cubes

1–2 tsp fructose

ACCEPTABLE FOR
 RAPID WEIGHT LOSS
and

 WEIGHT CONTROL

1 Preheat the oven to 350°F. Lightly butter a baking dish large enough to hold the chicken.

2 Rinse the chicken breasts with cold water and pat dry with paper towels. Place each breast between 2 pieces of heavy plastic wrap or parchment paper. Using a rolling pin, pound each breast to flatten to an even thickness of about ¼-inch. Remove the top layer of plastic wrap.

3 Place a few slices of fig down the center of each, and fold in the sides to make a package. Drizzle with a little olive oil and season with salt. Secure each package with a toothpick or small skewer, and lay inside the dish, seam-side down.

4 Scatter the shallots over the top, and pour in the white wine. Cover with foil and bake 20 minutes, until chicken is white throughout, but still juicy. Remove the chicken from the dish and keep warm. Gradually whisk the butter into the cooking juices until it has emulsified into a sauce. Keep warm.

6 For the garnish, increase the oven temperature to 400°F. Cut a cross in the top of the remaining 4 figs. Pinch the bottom of each fig to force open the top, then place on a baking sheet. Sprinkle with the fructose and drizzle with a little olive oil. Roast 5 minutes, until just softened.

7 To serve, place a chicken package on each of 4 warmed serving plates. Spoon the sauce on top, and garnish each plate with a roasted whole fig. Serve at once.

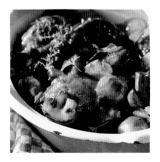

Coq au vin

Coq au vin is such a classic that it can sometimes be overlooked. Although it is not a 'one-pot' dish, its preparation is not as complicated as it might appear at first glance. Best of all, the results are well worth it.

SERVES 4

PREPARATION TIME
30 minutes

COOKING TIME
1¼ hours

INGREDIENTS
1 whole chicken, about 3 lb, cut into serving pieces
1 bottle dry red wine
pinch of salt
olive oil
6 oz pearl or small "boiling" onions, soaked in hot water until softened, then peeled
1 tbsp butter
1 tbsp finely chopped fresh thyme leaves
1 bay leaf (fresh is best)
2 cups beef stock
¼ lb thick-sliced bacon, cut crosswise into ¼-in pieces or pancetta, chopped
1½ cups mushrooms, chopped
2 tbsp chopped fresh parsley

ACCEPTABLE FOR
 RAPID WEIGHT LOSS
and

 WEIGHT CONTROL

1 Place the chicken pieces in a large, heavy duty zipper-lock bag. Pour in ¾ cup of wine, and seal closed. Marinate in the refrigerator, turning several times to redistribute the wine, for at least 1 hour or as long as overnight.

2 Transfer the chicken to a clean work surface. Discard the marinade. Season chicken with salt and drizzle with olive oil. Heat a large, heavy-bottomed Dutch oven over high heat, add the chicken, and cook for 6–7 minutes, turning until golden on all sides.

3 Remove chicken from the pan and pat dry with paper towels. Wipe the pan clean and set aside.

4 Place the pearl onions in a skillet, cover with water, and add the butter. Cook over high heat, stirring occasionally, until the water evaporates and the onions are browned.

5 Combine the onions, thyme, and bay leaf in the Dutch oven. Add the remaining 2½ cups of wine and the stock. Return the chicken to the pan and bring to a boil. Reduce heat to low and cook, covered, about 40 minutes, or until cooked through. Remove the chicken from the pan and keep warm. Cook over high heat, uncovered, until the liquid is reduced by ⅓.

6 Meanwhile, fry the bacon in a skillet over high heat for 2–3 minutes until crispy. Remove to a plate. Add 1 tablespoon of oil and cook mushrooms until lightly browned, about 5 minutes.

7 Pour the reduced sauce over the chicken. Stir in the onions, bacon, and mushroom, and sprinkle over the parsley. Serve at once.

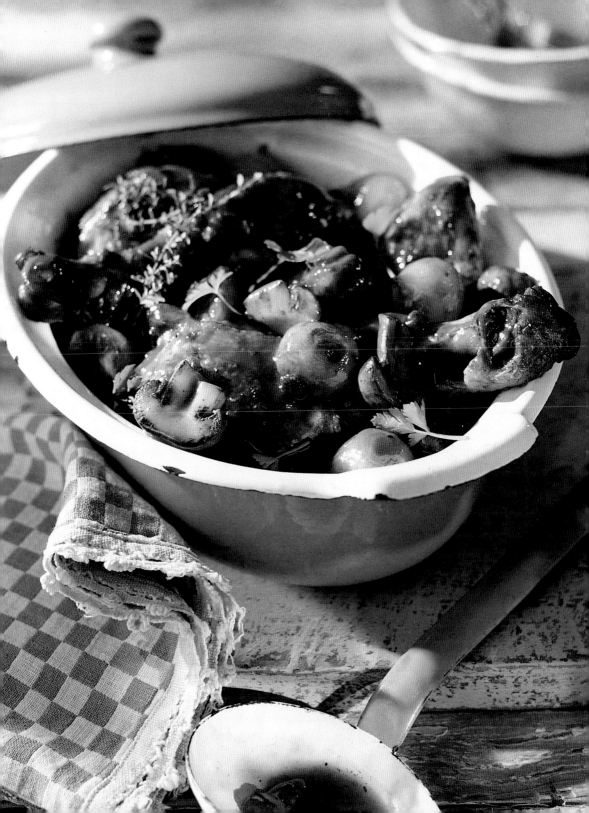

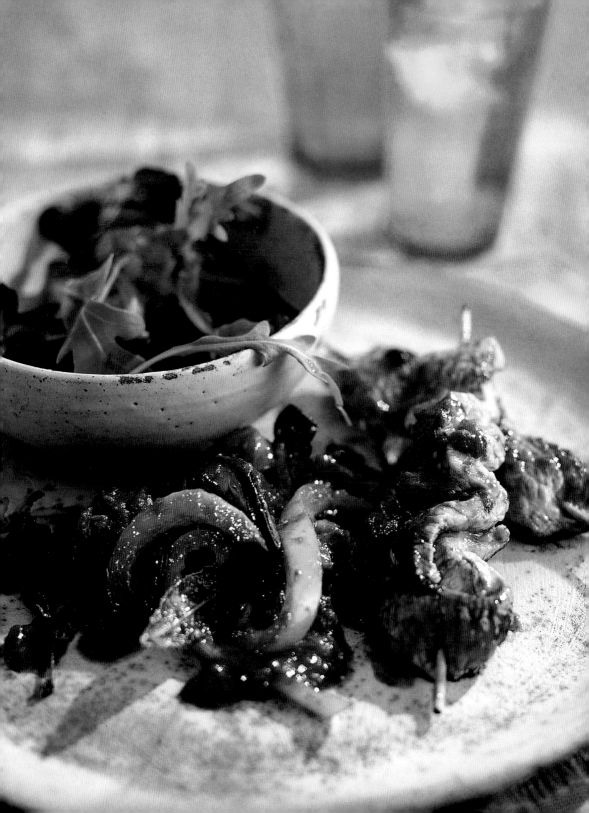

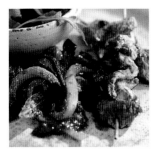

Turkey brochettes with vegetables à la provençal

This dish reveals its provençal roots in the tomatoes, eggplant, and bell peppers used in the sauce. Strong, earthy flavors are trademarks of provençal cuisine, with the emphasis on using the best possible ingredients for the best possible result.

SERVES 4

PREPARATION TIME
25 minutes

COOKING TIME
25 minutes

INGREDIENTS
4 turkey cutlets, about 4oz each, cut into thick slices

Olive oil

1 eggplant, cut into rounds about ¼ inch thick (If eggplant is large, cut the rounds in half.)

1 yellow bell pepper, seeded and cut into strips

1 tbsp dry white wine or vermouth

1 (14½ ounce) can diced tomatoes

1½ tbsp fresh thyme leaves

1 or 2 bay leaves (fresh is best)

ACCEPTABLE FOR
  RAPID WEIGHT LOSS
and

  WEIGHT CONTROL

1 To make the brochettes: Divide the turkey into 4 strips and thread 2 pieces onto each of 8 skewers. (If using wooden or bamboo skewers, these should be soaked in water for at least 15 minutes before using, to prevent burning.)

2 Heat 3 tablespoons olive oil in a large skillet over a high heat. Cook the brochettes for 5 minutes, turning frequently to brown all sides. Remove from the pan and set aside–but do not remove the meat from the skewers.

3 Add the eggplant and bell pepper to the same pan, adding more oil as needed, and cook for 7-9 minutes, stirring occasionally, until the vegetables are softened and the eggplant is starting to brown.

4 Add the wine, tomatoes, thyme, and bay leaf. Reduce the heat to medium and cook for 5 minutes, stirring occasionally to blend flavors.

5 Return the turkey brochettes to the pan and cook until heated through and meat is white throughout, 3 to 6 minutes. Add salt and freshly ground black pepper to taste, and discard the bay leaf.

6 To serve, place the turkey brochettes, still on their skewers, on a warmed serving platter alongside the vegetables. Serve at once.

Braised lamb shanks

SERVES 4

PREPARATION TIME
15 minutes, plus 24 hours
for marinating

COOKING TIME
2½ hours

INGREDIENTS
4 lamb shanks, 14 oz each
1 bottle dry red wine plus
1 onion, chopped
1 bunch of fresh thyme, plus
extra for garnish
1 bay leaf
1 qt veal or beef stock

ACCEPTABLE FOR

RAPID WEIGHT LOSS
and

WEIGHT CONTROL

Lamb shanks benefit greatly from long, slow cooking. The flavor becomes mellow, and the meat will be so tender it falls off the bone. You will also find that marinating the shanks prior to cooking is definitely worth the effort.

1 Place the lamb shanks in a large, heavy-duty zipper-lock bag. Pour in 1½ cups of wine and seal to close. Marinate in the refrigerator, turning several times to redistribute the wine, at least 24 hours or as long as 48 hours. Pat dry with paper towels.

2 Heat 2 tablespoons olive oil in a Dutch oven over medium-high heat. Working in batches if necessary, cook the lamb shanks without crowding until nicely browned on all sides, about 12 minutes. Transfer lamb shanks to a plate and discard the fat that remains in the Dutch oven. (Do not wash.)

3 In the same pot, heat 1 tablespoon olive oil over medium heat. Add onion and cook, stirring occasionally, until softened but not browned, 3 to 5 minutes. Pour in the remaining 1½ cups wine and the stock. Bring to a boil, scraping up any browned bits that cling to the bottom of the pot. Add the lamb shanks, thyme, and bay leaf. Cook, covered, over medium heat, 2 hours or until tender.

4 Using a slotted spoon, transfer lamb shanks to a large, warmed platter and cover loosely with aluminum foil. Bring the liquid remaining in the Dutch oven to a boil over high heat. Cook, stirring occasionally, until the liquid has reduced by ⅓ Remove the bay leaf (and the thyme sprigs, if desired) and skim off the fat. Spoon sauce over the lamb shanks. Garnish with fresh thyme and serve warm.

North African lamb stew

SERVES 4

PREPARATION TIME
35 minutes

COOKING TIME
1½ hours

INGREDIENTS
3 tbsp coriander seed
3 tbsp cumin seed
3 tbsp fennel seed
1 tsp hot red pepper flakes
olive oil
2¼ lb boneless leg of lamb or lean lamb shoulder, trimmed of any fat or gristle and cut into 2¼-in cubes
3 onions, sliced
1 tbsp minced fresh ginger
1 tsp paprika
½ cup (3½ oz) tomato purée
½ cup (3½ oz) veal or beef stock
½ cup (3½ oz) cooked chickpeas
1½ lb eggplant, cut into ¼-in dice
4 large tomatoes
1 tbsp chopped fresh cilantro

ACCEPTABLE FOR

RAPID WEIGHT LOSS
and

WEIGHT CONTROL

This stew is actually a braise—where the meat is cooked slowly in very little liquid. Not only is this a common method of cooking in North Africa, but the flavors are also typical of its cuisines.

1 Roast coriander seed, cumin seed, fennel seed, and pepper flakes in a dry skillet over medium heat, stirring until fragrant, about 1 minute. Grind to a powder using a mortar and pestle or electric spice mill.

2 Season the lamb with salt. Heat 2 tablespoons olive oil in a large, heavy-bottomed saucepan over medium heat. Working in batches, cook the lamb, turning, until nicely browned on all sides. Drain the lamb in a colander placed over a bowl to catch the juices. Add onions to the same pot, and cook until softened and golden in color, 5 to 9 minutes. Transfer to the colander with the lamb. Finally, add the ginger to the pan and cook, stirring, just until fragrant, 1 to 2 minutes. Turn the contents of the colander and the juice from the bowl beneath it back into the pan. Add the ground spices, paprika, salt to taste, tomato purée, and stock. Bring to a boil. Reduce heat to low and cook, covered, 1½ hours, or until meat is tender. Stir in the chickpeas and cook until heated.

3 Toward the end of the cooking time, preheat the oven to 475°F. Place the eggplant on a large baking sheet, drizzle with olive oil, and sprinkle with salt. Roast 15 to 20 minutes, or until golden brown.

4 To blanch the tomatoes, plunge into boiling water for 30 seconds to 1 minute, then refresh in ice water for another minute. Peel, quarter, and remove the seeds, reserving the juice. Cut tomatoes into strips. Pour tomato juices back into the stew.

5 When the lamb is fork-tender, skim off any fat that has risen to the top. Stir in the cilantro. Turn the stew into a shallow serving bowl. Scatter the eggplant and tomato strips over the top. Serve warm.

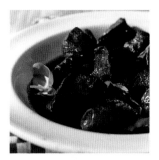

Lamb provençal

Canned tomato purée is used in the base for the stew; sweet and juicy oven-roasted cherry tomatoes and fresh basil are added to provide a burst of fresh flavor

SERVES 4

PREPARATION TIME
20 minutes

COOKING TIME
50 minutes

INGREDIENTS

2¼ lb boneless leg of lamb, trimmed of any fat or gristle and cut into 1-in cubes

olive oil

1 white onion, finely chopped

1 tbsp good-quality herbes de Provence, plus 1 tsp for sprinkling

¼ cup dry red wine

1 can (14½ oz) tomato purée

1 cup veal or beef stock

1 cup cherry tomatoes

3 tbsp fresh basil leaves, shredded or torn

ACCEPTABLE FOR

RAPID WEIGHT LOSS
and

WEIGHT CONTROL

1   Season lamb with salt. In a heavy-bottomed Dutch oven, heat 2 tablespoons olive oil over medium-heat. Working in batches, cook the lamb until nicely browned on all sides. Remove with a slotted spoon and place in a large colander placed over a bowl to catch the meat juices.

2   Add the onion to the pot, adding more olive oil if needed. Cook, stirring, until softened and browned, 3 to 5 minutes. Stir in the reserved lamb and its juices, the wine, 1 tablespoon herbes de Provence, tomato purée, and stock. Bring to a boil over medium-high heat. Reduce heat to medium-low and cook, partially covered, until lamb is fork-tender, about 45 minutes. Skim off any fat that has risen to the top.

3   To prepare the tomatoes, preheat the oven to 400°F. Place the tomatoes on a baking sheet in a roasting pan and drizzle with olive oil. Sprinkle them with salt and the remaining teaspoon herbes de Provence. Roast 4 to 5 minutes, until the tomato skins blister and crack. Keep warm.

4   When the lamb is tender, turn the stew into a shallow serving bowl. Scatter the cherry tomatoes and basil, and drizzle any of the tomato cooking juices over the top. Serve warm.

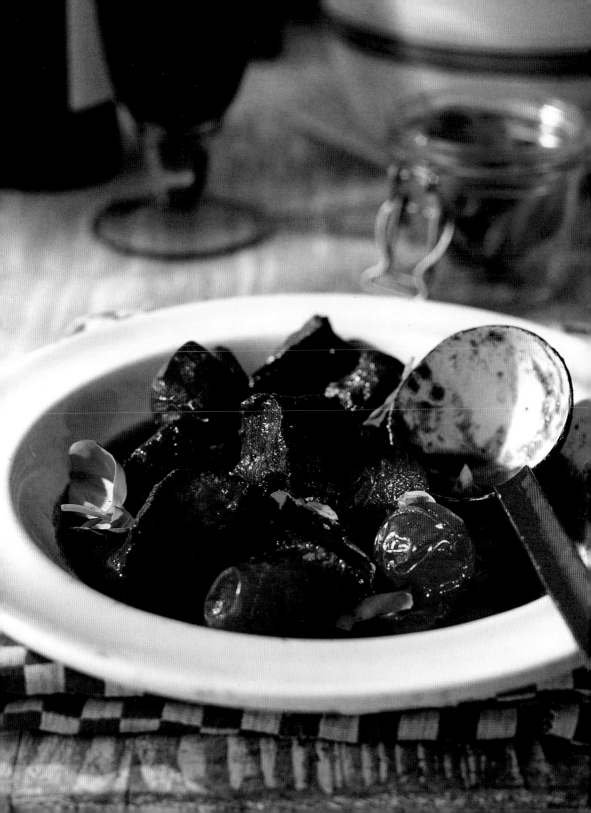

Entrecôte steaks Bordeaux style

SERVES 4

PREPARATION TIME
25 minutes

COOKING TIME
10 minutes

INGREDIENTS
1 tsp butter
6 shallots, finely chopped
1½ cups dry red wine
3½ tbsp red wine vinegar
1 cup beef stock
4 rib-eye steaks, each cut
into 1½ to 2-in thick, trimmed
of any excess fat
salt and freshly ground
pepper
olive oil
¼ lb fresh porcini or other
meaty wild mushrooms,
trimmed and sliced
1 tbsp chopped fresh parsley

ACCEPTABLE FOR
  RAPID WEIGHT LOSS
and

  WEIGHT CONTROL

Entrecôte is a thick steak cut from between the ninth and eleventh ribs—hardly surprising, as *entrecôte* is French for 'between the ribs'. Supremely tender, this type of steak responds best to cooking.

1 To prepare the red wine sauce, heat a heavy-bottomed saucepan over medium heat. Add the butter and shallots. Cook, covered, 1 to 2 minutes, or until softened. Add the wine and red wine vinegar. Bring to a boil and cook uncovered to reduce the liquid by ⅔. Add the stock and continue boiling until the sauce is thick enough to coat the back of a spoon, 5 to 10 minutes. Remove from the heat, add salt to taste, and keep warm.

2 Working in batches if necessary, heat 1 or 2 heavy-bottomed skillets over medium-high heat. Add enough olive oil to lightly coat the bottom of the skillet(s). When hot, add steaks without crowding. Cook, turning once, until steaks are nicely browned on the outside, 6 to 7 minutes per side for medium-rare. As steaks are done, transfer to a warmed plastic or carving board to rest 5 to 10 minutes. Cover loosely with foil to keep warm.

3 Reduce the heat under the pan to medium, and add the mushrooms. Cook briskly for about 3 minutes, then add the red wine sauce, stirring to deglaze the pan. Remove from the heat and keep warm.

4 To serve, place a steak on each of 4 warmed dinner plates. Spoon the red wine sauce with mushrooms over the top. Sprinkle with parsley. Serve at once.

Daube de boeuf

SERVES 4

PREPARATION TIME
30 minutes, plus at least
12 hours for marinating

COOKING TIME
3 hours

INGREDIENTS

3 lb boneless beef chuck, cut into 1-in cubes

1 large onion, thinly sliced

2 garlic cloves, finely chopped

zest of 1 orange, cut into strips

1 bunch of fresh thyme (about 2 tbsp leaves)

sprig of fresh rosemary, a couple of sprigs of parsley and a bay leaf tied together with cotton twine

2 cups dry red wine

1 tbsp olive oil

¼ lb thick-sliced bacon cut crosswise into ¼-in pieces

3 celery ribs

1 cup beef stock

¼ cup kalamata olives, pitted

ACCEPTABLE FOR
 RAPID WEIGHT LOSS
and

 WEIGHT CONTROL

Daubes are common throughout France, as yet another slow-cooking method to make meat as tender as possible. A heavy clay pot known as a *daubière* is often used when making this, but any deep, flameproof casserole with a lid will do.

1 Put the beef cubes in a large, heavy duty zipper-lock bag. Pour in 1 cup of wine, half the onion, half the garlic, half the orange zest, and half the thyme. Seal to close. Marinate in the refrigerator, turning several times to redistribute the ingredients, for at least 12 or up to 24 hours.

2 Preheat the oven to 325°F. Drain the beef, discarding the marinade. Pat dry with paper towels. Heat the olive oil in a large, deep, flameproof or Dutch oven casserole over medium heat. Add the bacon and cook, stirring occasionally, until nicely browned, 5 to 7 minutes. Remove with a slotted spoon and set aside.

3 Increase heat to medium-high. Working in batches, cook the beef until nicely browned on all sides. Remove with a slotted spoon and place in a large colander situated over a bowl to catch the juices.

4 In the same pot, combine the remaining onion and celery. Cook over medium heat, stirring occasionally, until vegetables are softened but not browned, 3 to 5 minutes. Stir in the garlic, the remaining thyme, and orange zest. Add the remaining 1 cup of wine and the stock. Bring to a boil, scraping up any browned bits from the bottom of the pan. Add the beef, its juices, and the reserved bacon.

5 Place a sheet of parchment paper over the top of the casserole then cover with the lid. Cook, covered, 2 to 2½ hours, or until meat is fork-tender. Remove the lid and paper, and skim off any fat. Stir in the olives. Cook over high heat until the liquid has thickened, 5 to 10 minutes. Serve warm, spooned into shallow bowls.

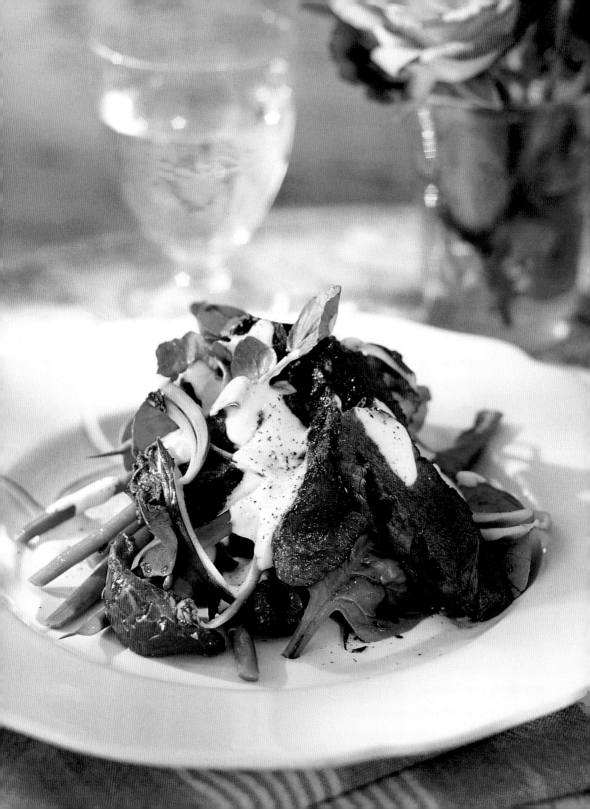

Grilled beef with spinach and horseradish sauce

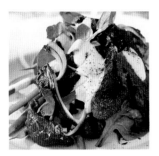

SERVES 4

PREPARATION TIME
30 minutes

COOKING TIME
15 minutes

INGREDIENTS
½ lb thin green beans or haricots vert, trimmed

1 boneless top round steak cut about 1-in thick

1 red onion, halved
olive oil

2 cups baby spinach leaves

1 bunch watercress

½ cup sun-dried tomato halves, coarsely chopped

HORSERADISH DRESSING
½ cup plain yogurt, preferably Greek-style
1 tbsp creamed horseradish

2 tbsp lemon juice

2 tbsp heavy (whipping) cream

2 garlic cloves, crushed through a press

2 or 3 drops of Tabasco, or to taste

salt and freshly ground black pepper

ACCEPTABLE FOR
   RAPID WEIGHT LOSS
and .

   WEIGHT CONTROL

Few can resist succulent slices of grilled beef served with a fresh salad. The horseradish dressing is made memorable with a kick of tangy lemon and a fiery hint of Tabasco.

1 Fit a metal steamer basket inside a medium saucepan. Add an inch of water and bring to a boil over high heat. Reduce heat to low, add green beans, and cover. Cook until beans are crisp-tender, 3 to 4 minutes. Set aside.

2 Preheat an indoor or outdoor grill. When it is hot, brush the steak and the onion with olive oil. Season with salt and pepper. Grill the meat for 4 minutes on each side for medium-rare. Let rest for at least 5 minutes. Meanwhile, grill the onion, 3 minutes per side.

3 Combine the spinach, watercress, sun-dried tomatoes, and reserved beans. Toss gently to mix, then arrange on a serving platter.

4 To make the horseradish dressing, combine the yogurt, horseradish, lemon juice, cream, garlic, Tabasco, salt, and freshly ground black pepper to taste in a small bowl. Stir to blend well. Taste, adding more seasonings as needed.

5 Cut the beef into thin diagonal slices and arrange over the salad. Thinly slice the onion and scatter over the top. Drizzle with horseradish dressing and serve at once.

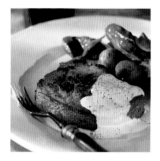

SERVES 4

PREPARATION TIME
20 minutes

COOKING TIME
20 minutes

INGREDIENTS
4 boneless veal loin chops,
cut about 1-in thick (about
6 oz each)

olive oil

salt and freshly ground black
pepper

GORGONZOLA SAUCE
4 tbsp heavy (whipping)
cream

2 tbsp veal or beef stock

1½ tbsp sherry vinegar

3 tbsp dry sherry

½ cup crumbled Gorgonzola
cheese

ACCEPTABLE FOR
  RAPID WEIGHT LOSS
and

  WEIGHT CONTROL

Veal chops in Gorgonzola sauce

Slightly pungent Gorgonzola makes a worthy partner for elegant veal chops. Best of all, dinner is really ready in less than an hour.

1 To make the sauce: In a small, heavy-bottomed saucepan, combine 1 tablespoon of the cream, stock, sherry vinegar, and sherry to a boil over medium heat. Reduce heat to low and cook, uncovered, until the sauce is reduced to ⅔ of its original volume. Preheat the oven to 400°F.

2 Whisk in the Gorgonzola a few pieces at a time, then add the whipped cream and stir through gently. Set aside to keep warm. In a small bowl, whisk the remaining 3 tablespoons cream until soft peaks form. Fold into the Gorgonzola sauce and keep warm.

3 Season the chops with salt and pepper. Working in batches if necessary, add enough oil to coat the bottom of a large skillet over medium-high heat. Add chops without crowding and cook, turning once, until nicely browned on the outside, 2 to 3 minutes. Reduce heat to medium and continue cooking, turning once again, until meat reaches desired doneness (about another 6 minutes per side for medium). Transfer cooked chops to a carving board to rest 5 to 10 minutes before serving.

4 Cut chops into thick slices, or leave whole. Divide veal among 4 warmed serving plates. Drizzle Gorgonzola sauce over each and serve at once.

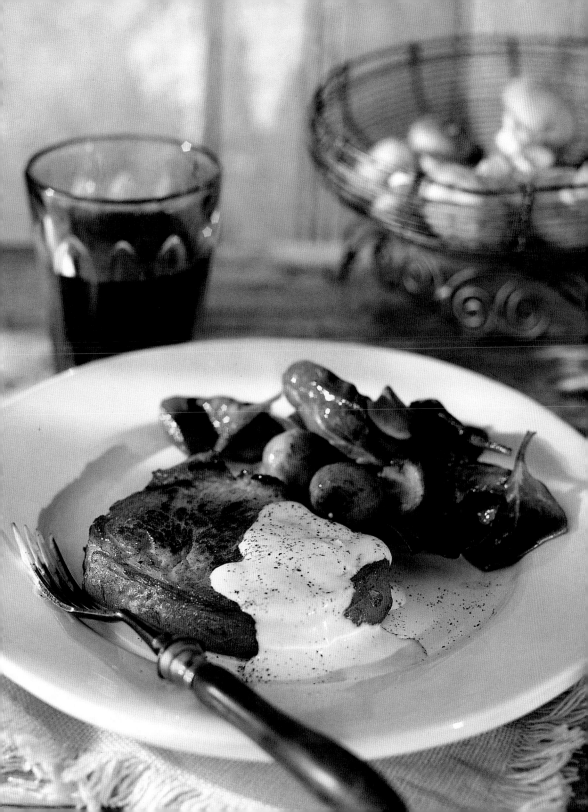

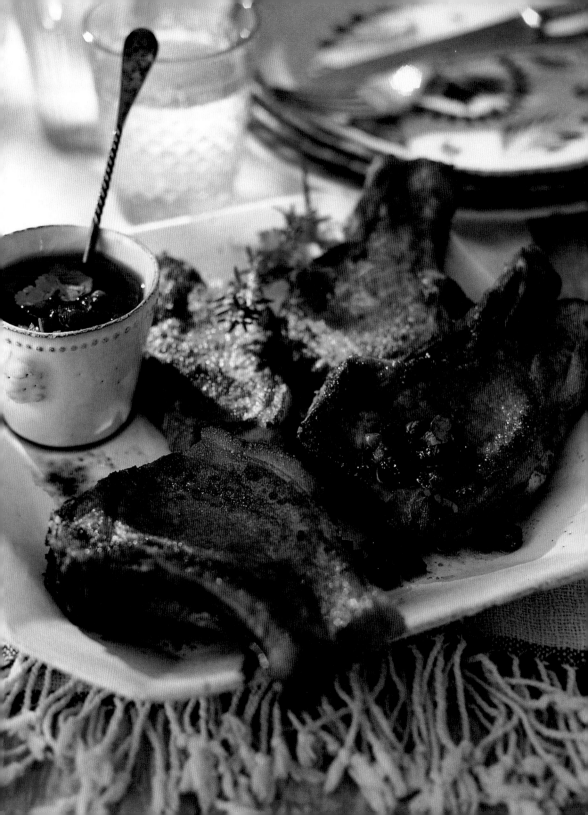

Pork chops in caper sauce

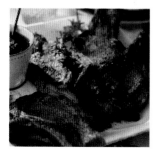

A simple dry rub adds extra zing to these pork chops. The finishing touch is a piquant sauce bursting with the flavor of capers, tomato, lemon, and parsley.

SERVES 4

PREPARATION TIME
20 minutes

COOKING TIME
10 minutes

INGREDIENTS
2 tbsp almond powder or ground almonds
1 tsp paprika
½ tsp salt
½ tsp cracked black pepper
olive oil
4 bone-in pork rib chops, cut about 1-in thick
8 capers to garnish

CAPER SAUCE
1 very ripe tomato, halved, seeded, and diced
1 tbsp capers, rinsed and drained
2 tbsp chopped fresh parsley
3 tbsp olive oil
juice of 1 lemon

ACCEPTABLE FOR
RAPID WEIGHT LOSS
and
WEIGHT CONTROL

1 Mix together the almond powder, paprika, salt, and pepper in a shallow bowl or on a plate. Coat pork chops in this mixture on both sides.

2 Working in batches if necessary, heat 1 tablespoon olive oil in a skillet over medium-high heat. When hot, cook the chops until nicely browned on both sides. Reduce heat to medium-low and continue cooking until meat is white throughout, about 10 minutes total.

3 To make the caper sauce, combine the tomato, capers, parsley, olive oil, and lemon juice. Stir to mix. Add salt and freshly ground black pepper to taste.

4 Place a pork chop on each of 4 warmed plates, and top each serving with a spoonful of the caper sauce. Garnish with capers and serve at once.

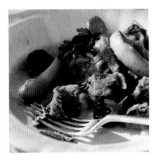

SERVES 4

COOKING TIME
45 minutes, plus at least
1 hour for marinating

INGREDIENTS
olive oil

2¼ lb lean boneless pork, cut
into ½-in cubes

2 tsp dry white wine

2 tsp white wine vinegar

a few whole black
peppercorns

2 bay leaves (fresh is best)

1 celeriac bulb (celery root),
peeled and diced

3 leeks, cut into rings

1 onion, chopped

1 cup chicken stock

3 or 4 apples, cut into
6 wedges

2 tbsp fructose

1 tbsp butter

½ cup pitted prunes

1 tsp lemon juice

1 tsp Dijon mustard

2 tbsp chopped fresh parsley

ACCEPTABLE FOR
RAPID WEIGHT LOSS
and

WEIGHT CONTROL

Pork with apples and prunes

This dish is similar to a fricassée, but at the end of cooking, the vegetables with which the meat is stewed are blended to make a smooth sauce. The final touch is a topping of caramelized apples and prunes, for contrasting sweetness.

1 Put the pork in a large, zipper-lock plastic bag with the white wine, vinegar, peppercorns, and 1 bay leaf. Marinate in the refrigerator for at least 1 hour, preferably overnight, turning the bag once or twice to redistribute the ingredients.

2 Drain pork, discarding marinade. Pat dry. Heat 1 tablespoon oil in a heavy-bottomed skillet over medium–high heat. Working in batches if necessary, cook pork, turning, until nicely browned on all sides, about 10 minutes. Transfer pork to a plate.

3 Reduce the heat to medium. Using the same pan, cook the celeriac, leek, and onion for 3 to 5 minutes, stirring, until softened. Add 1 bay leaf and the stock and bring to a boil. Return the pork to the pan, cover with a lid, and reduce heat to medium-low. Cook 40 minutes longer, stirring from time to time, until meat is tender.

4 Place the apple segments in large frying pan over a high heat. Add the fructose and the tablespoon of butter. Cook the apples for 6 minutes, until slightly browned at the edges, then add the prunes. Keep warm until needed.

5 Remove the pork from the vegetables and reserve. Discard the bay leaf. Blend or process the vegetable mixture (including the liquid) for a few minutes, until smooth. Return to the pan to reheat.

6 Stir the meat into the sauce. Turn mixture into a warmed dish to serve. Top with the caramelized apples and prunes. Sprinkle with parsley and serve warm.

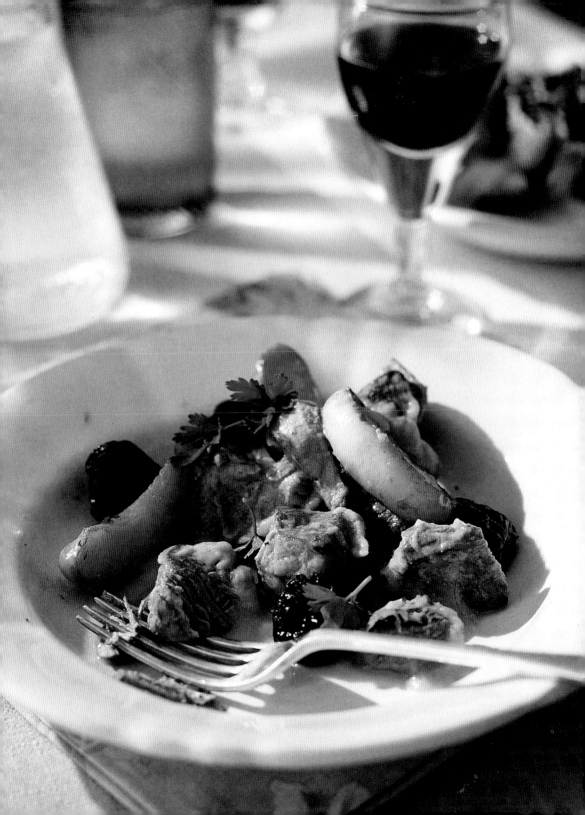

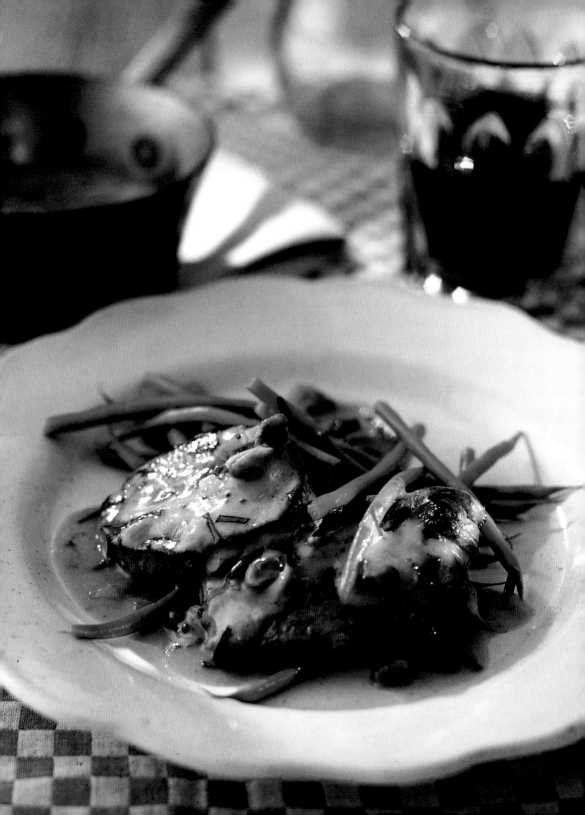

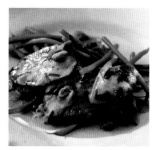

SERVES 4

PREPARATION TIME
20 minutes

COOKING TIME
25 minutes

INGREDIENTS
2 tsp rinsed and drained capers

olive oil

5 shallots, finely chopped

1½ tbsp white wine

1 cup veal or beef stock

1 cup crème fraîche or sour cream

1 tsp coarse-grain mustard

½ tsp Dijon mustard

½ bunch of chopped fresh tarragon or chives

1 tbsp goose fat or olive oil

4 boneless pork chops or pork tenderloins, cut about ½-in thick

ACCEPTABLE FOR
RAPID WEIGHT LOSS
and
WEIGHT CONTROL

Pork with herbed mustard

A creamy, herb-infused mustard sauce is just the thing to smother thick, succulent pork chops. The pork is cooked in a touch of goose fat to help the meat retain its moisture, but you can substitute olive oil if you prefer.

1 Heat 2 tablespoons olive oil in a small saucepan over medium-high heat. Add the shallot, white wine, capers, and stock. Bring to a boil, then continue cooking 12 to 15 minutes, until the liquid is about ⅓ of its original volume.

2 Reduce heat to low. Whisk in the crème fraîche, then add the coarse and Dijon mustards. Stir in the tarragon. Keep warm.

3 Meanwhile, heat a large skillet over medium heat. Melt the goose fat in the pan. Working in batches if necessary, add the pork. Cook the meat 3 to 4 minutes on each side, until golden on the outside and white throughout.

4 Drain the chops on paper towels to absorb any excess fat. Place a chop on each of 4 warmed plates and spoon mustard sauce over the top. Serve at once.

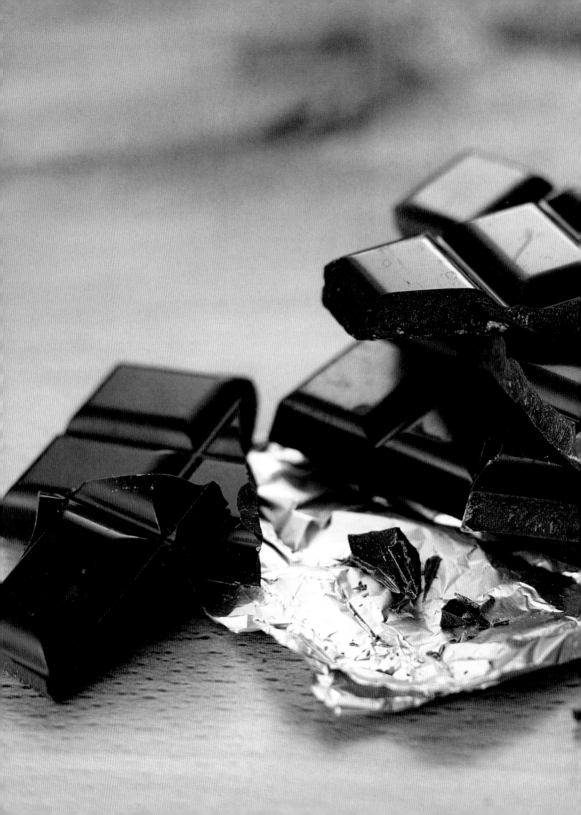

Desserts

All of the desserts in this chapter are acceptable as part of the Rapid Weight Loss Plan and the Weight Control Plan. The decadent Chocolate cake (*see pp232-33*) is a favorite low–GI treat at the Montignac Boutique & Café in London. Now, for the first time, the Café shares its popular recipes so you, too, can enjoy delicious, guilt-free desserts at home.

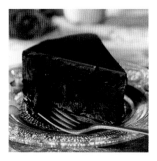

SERVES 6–8

PREPARATION TIME
30 minutes, plus overnight refrigeration

COOKING TIME
15 minutes

INGREDIENTS
11 oz dark chocolate (70% cocoa solids), broken into pieces, plus extra 6½ oz for topping
10 large eggs, separated

ACCEPTABLE FOR
  RAPID WEIGHT LOSS
and

  WEIGHT CONTROL

Chocolate cake

This cake shows the benefit of using high-quality ingredients—in this case, chocolate. The secret is to have your oven as hot as possible and to work quickly once the chocolate has melted. The result is a rich but not overpowering delight.

1 Line the bottom and sides of an 8-inch round springform pan with baking parchment. (The collar lining the side of the tin should rise above the top of the pan.) Preheat the oven to 500°F.

2 Place a large, clean, heatproof dry bowl over a saucepan of barely simmering water, making sure the bowl does not touch the water. Place the chocolate in the bowl. Stir occasionally until melted and smooth, about 10 minutes.

3 Put the egg whites in a large bowl, and, using a hand-held electric mixer, beat until stiff peaks form. Do not overbeat.

4 Remove the melted chocolate from the pan and let cool 5 minutes. Gently stir together the beaten egg yolks and add to the melted chocolate. Add a couple of tablespoons of the beaten egg white and stir just to combine. Quickly and gently fold in the rest of the egg white until the mixture has the consistency of a soufflé or light mousse. Do not overmix.

5 Pour the chocolate mixture into the pan and bake for 8 minutes exactly. Remove the pan from the oven and let cool 30 minutes; then refrigerate, covered, 12 hours or overnight.

6 To finish, take the cake out of the refrigerator and turn it onto a large plate or a piece of wax paper on a flat work surface. Melt the extra chocolate as described in step 2. Pour a thin film of chocolate over the cake. Chill in the refrigerator 15 minutes. To serve, dip a sharp knife in hot water and use to slice the cake.

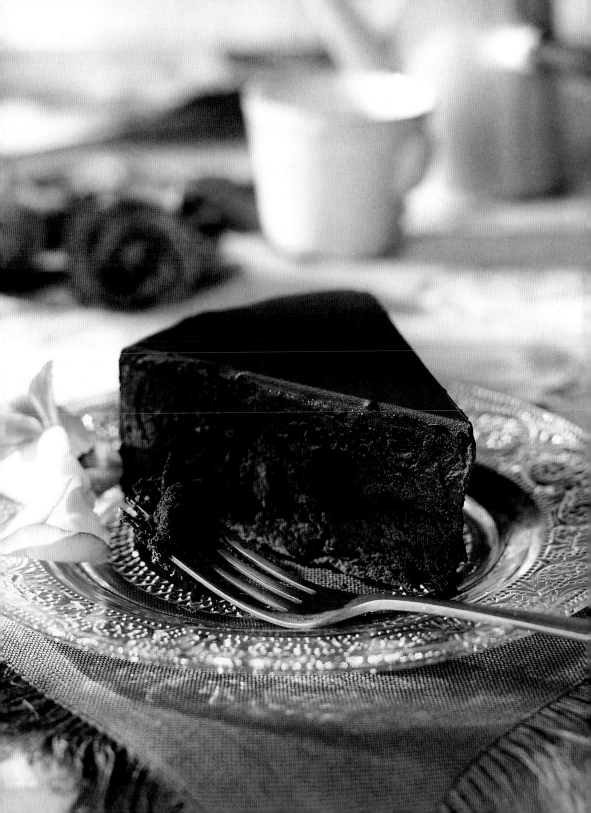

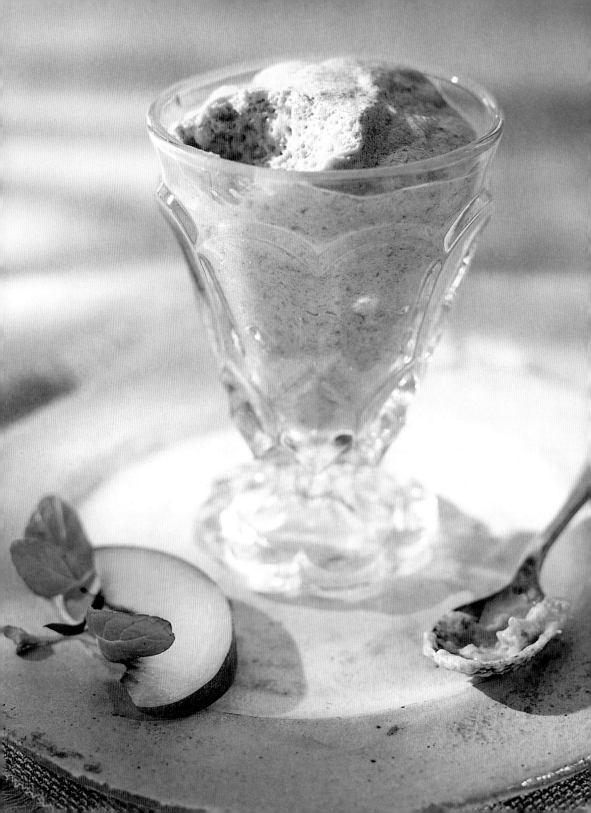

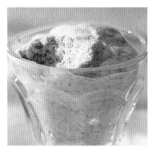

Peach mousse

Choose the ripest, sweetest, and most fragrant peaches you can find for this light and fluffy mousse—but watch out for bruising. For the best appearance, it is better to choose a peach variety with colored, rather than white, flesh.

SERVES 4

PREPARATION TIME
40 minutes

COOKING TIME
5 minutes

INGREDIENTS
1⅛ tsp unflavored gelatin (half of a ¼ oz package)

1 lb peaches, peeled, cored and quartered

2 oz fructose plus a little extra for sweetening

juice of ½ lemon

2 eggs, separated

1 tbsp heavy (whipping) cream

1 tsp vanilla extract

ACCEPTABLE FOR
  RAPID WEIGHT LOSS
and

  WEIGHT CONTROL

1 Soak the gelatin in cold water until softened, about 5 minutes.

2 In a food processor, blend the peaches with half the fructose and the lemon juice.

3 Beat the egg yolks in a heatproof bowl with the remaining fructose until light and fluffy. Heat gently over a saucepan of barely simmering water, until the fructose has dissolved and the mixture coats the back of a spoon. Remove the bowl from the heat and stir in the gelatin. Let cool briefly.

4 Whisk together the egg yolk mixture and the peach mixture.

5 Whisk the egg whites until stiff peaks form. (Alternatively, beat with clean beaters in an electric mixer.) In a separate small bowl, whip the cream until firm, adding the vanilla extract and a little extra fructose to sweeten slightly.

6 Gently fold the cream into the peach mixture, then, using a large rubber spatula, gently fold in the egg whites, ⅓ at a time, using a spatula—do not stir as you want to keep as much air as possible in the mixture.

7 Pour mousse mixture into parfait glasses or small ramekins. Cover and refrigerate at least 4 hours before serving.

Chocolate vanilla pots

SERVES 4

PREPARATION TIME
25 minutes, plus 10 or so
hours for chilling

COOKING TIME
15 minutes

INGREDIENTS

CHOCOLATE MOUSSE
1 cup heavy (whipping)
cream
1 cup milk
9 oz dark semisweet or
bittersweet chocolate (70%
cocoa solids), chopped
2 large eggs, beaten

VANILLA CREAM
2 cups heavy (whipping)
cream
9 large egg yolks
2 oz fructose
1 vanilla bean, pod split
lengthwise

Whipped cream to decorate
Chocolate flakes to decorate

ACCEPTABLE FOR
  RAPID WEIGHT LOSS
and

  WEIGHT CONTROL

These individual desserts look very tempting with their layers of chocolate and vanilla—and they are all the more tempting on the palate. If you have extra mousse after filling your serving glasses, simply make up another pot to enjoy later.

1 To make the chocolate mousse, place the chocolate in a blender or food processor. Combine with the cream and milk in a small, heavy-bottomed saucepan. Bring to a boil carefully—do not scorch.

2 When the cream mixture has just come to a boil, turn on the blender or processor, and slowly pour in the hot cream mixture. Add the eggs one at a time and blend until smooth. Divide mixture equally between 4 large parfait glasses or ramekins. (Mixture should fill only half the container.) Cover with plastic wrap and refrigerate 8 hours to set.

3 To make the vanilla cream, pour the cream into a medium, heavy-bottomed saucepan. Use the tip of a sharp knife to scrape the seeds from the vanilla pod into the cream. Over low heat, warm the mixture to just below a boil.

4 Meanwhile, put the egg yolks into a bowl and whisk in the fructose. Add some of the warm cream and quickly mix. Pour the egg mixture into the pan with the rest of the cream. Cook over low heat, stirring with a wooden spoon, until it thickens and coats the back of the spoon. Strain through a sieve and refrigerate for at least 2 hours.

5 When the chocolate mousse has set, pour the vanilla cream in on top. Fill the glasses almost to the rim, so that you have a layer of chocolate and a layer of vanilla cream. Chill until ready to serve.

6 Serve topped with a swirl of whipped cream and a sprinkle of shaved or grated chocolate.

Raspberry and chocolate mousse

SERVES 4

PREPARATION TIME
20 minutes, plus at least
4 hours for chilling

COOKING TIME
10 minutes

INGREDIENTS
5½ oz dark chocolate (70%
cocoa solids), broken into
pieces
1 tbsp heavy (whipping)
cream, at room temperature
1 cup raspberries, crushed
4 large eggs, separated

ACCEPTABLE FOR
 RAPID WEIGHT LOSS
and

 WEIGHT CONTROL

Chocolate and raspberries are an almost symbiotic pairing. Their flavors are set off well in this simple mousse. As with all mousses, the secret to the right result is to fold in the egg whites, not stir. The latter deflates the mousse.

1 Melt the chocolate in a bowl set over a saucepan of barely simmering water, making sure the bowl does not touch the water. Let cool and stir in the cream.

2 Beat the egg yolks and add to the chocolate mixture, then stir in the crushed raspberries.

3 Beat the egg whites until stiff peaks form. Gently fold into the chocolate mixture, ⅓ at a time, using a large spatula. Be careful not to overmix, as this will deflate the mousse.

4 Pour the mousse into a glass or ceramic serving dish, or just use 4 individual dishes. Refrigerate at least 4 hours or up to 24 hours before serving.

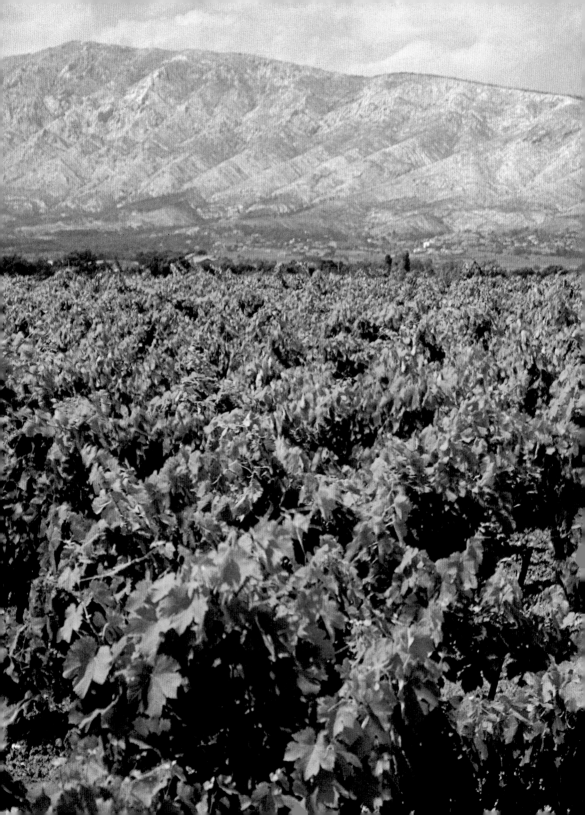

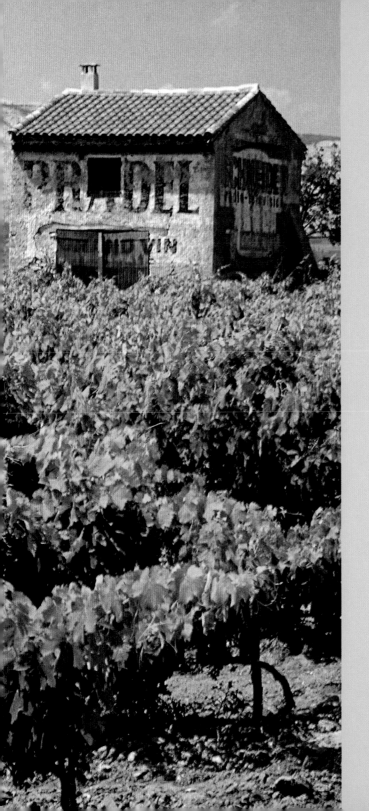

REFERENCE

GI chart: high to low

This glycemic index lists its entries from high to low. Use this chart to find out which foods have high GI values so that you can avoid them. Entries marked with an asterisk have a low concentration of carbohydrates (see p115), which means you can eat them in moderation on the Weight Control Plan.

Maltose (beer)	110	Cola drinks	70
Glucose (dextrose)	100	Cornflour	70
Potatoes (fried or french fried)	95	Potatoes (peeled; boiled)	70
Potatoes (peeled; baked)	95	Ravioli; tortellini	70
Rice (pre-cooked)	90	Rice (pre-cooked; long grain)	70
Puffed rice	85	Risotto rice	70
Honey	85	Sugar (sucrose)	70
Carrots (cooked)	85	Beets	65
Cornflakes	85	Brown flour	65
Flour, white bread	85	Corn (fresh; steamed)	65
Popcorn (no sugar added)	85	Couscous (cooked for five minutes)	65
Pretzels	85	Jam (with sugar)	65
Rice cakes	85	Orange juice (commercial variety)	65
Tapioca	85	Potatoes (baked; skin on)	65
Turnips*	85	Potatoes (boiled; skin on)	65
Crackers (made from white flour)	80	Raisins (dark or golden)	65
Potato chips	80	Sorbet (with sugar)	65
Potatoes (mashed)	80	Sultanas	65
Pumpkin*	75	Bananas	60
Watermelon*	75	Melon *	60
Cereals (refined)	70	Semolina (white, cooked)	60
Chocolate bar, milk chocolate	70	Rice (long grain; white)	60

Shortbread cookies	55	Apples (dried)	35
Butter cookies	55	Apricots (dried)	35
White pasta, soft-wheat (cooked well)	55	Beans, broad (peeled and cooked)	35
All-bran	50	Beans, haricot	35
Apple juice (fresh)	50	Figs (fresh)	35
Crêpes/pancakes (made with buckwheat)	50	Ice cream (made with alginates)	35
Kiwi	50	Kidney beans	35
Rice (unrefined Basmati)	50	Oranges	35
Rice (brown)	50	Natural (unflavored) yogurt	35
Sweet potatoes	50	Peas, dried (cooked)	35
Unrefined flour	50	Peas, fresh (cooked)	35
Buckwheat	45	Plums	35
Bulgur wheat (whole grain, cooked)	45	Prunes	35
Grapes (all kinds)	45	Quinoa	35
Orange juice (freshly squeezed)	45	Satsumas	35
Pasta (made from whole wheat flour)	45	Wild rice	35
Whole wheat bread with bran	45	Apples (fresh)	30
Black bread (German)	40	Apricots (fresh)	30
Figs (dried)	40	Beans, fresh green or string beans	30
Sorbet (sugarfree)	40	Carrots (raw)	30
Spaghetti, durum wheat (cooked *al dente*)	40	Chickpeas (garbanzo beans), cooked	30
Spaghetti, whole wheat (cooked *al dente*)	40	Garlic	30
Rye (whole wheat bread)	40	Grapefruit	30
Unrefined flour (bread)	40	Jam (sugarfree)	30
Unrefined flour (pasta)	40	Lentils (brown)	30

GI chart: alphabetical order

This glycemic index lists its entries in alphabetical order. Use this chart when you know the name of a carbohydrate, but don't know its GI value. Entries marked with an asterisk have a low concentration of carbohydrates (see p115), which means you can eat them in moderation on the Weight Control Plan.

All-bran	50	Buckwheat	45
Almonds; walnuts; hazelnuts	15	Bulgur wheat (whole grain, cooked)	45
Apples (dried)	35	Butter cookies	55
Apples (fresh)	30	Cabbage (all kinds)	15
Apple juice (fresh)	50	Carrots (cooked)*	85
Apricots (dried)	35	Carrots (raw)	30
Apricots (fresh)	30	Cauliflower	15
Artichokes	15	Celery	15
Asparagus	15	Celery root	15
Avocados	10	Cereals (refined)	70
Bananas	60	Cherries	25
Beans, broad (peeled and cooked)	35	Chickpeas (garbanzo beans), cooked	30
Beans, flageolet	25	Chinese vermicelli (soybean variety)	22
Beans, fresh green or string beans	30	Chocolate bar, milk chocolate	70
Beans, haricot	35	Cola drinks	70
Beets	65	Corn (fresh; steamed)	65
Blackberries	25	Cornflakes	85
Black bread (German)	40	Cornstarch	70
Brazil nuts	15	Couscous (cooked for five minutes)	65
Broccoli	15	Crêpes/pancakes (made with buckwheat)	50
Brown flour (brown bread)	65	Crackers (made from white flour)	80
Brussels sprouts	15	Cucumber	15

GI chart: high to low

Lentils (red)	30	Pumpkin seeds	15
Lentils (yellow)	30	Sunflower seeds	15
Milk (1% low-fat or skim)	30	Olives (all kinds)	15
Mung beans (soaked and cooked for 20 minutes)	30	Asparagus	15
Nectarines	30	Artichokes	15
Peaches	30	Broccoli	15
Pears	30	Brussels sprouts	15
Tomatoes	30	Cabbage (all kinds)	15
Beans, flageolet	25	Cauliflower	15
Cherries	25	Celery root	15
Dark chocolate (70 percent cocoa)	25	Celery	15
Lentils (green)	25	Cucumber	15
Strawberries	25	Fennel	15
Blackberries	25	Herbs	15
Raspberries	25	Leeks	15
Soybeans (cooked)	25	Lettuce (all kinds)	15
Split peas (yellow, cooked for 20 minutes)	25	Mushrooms	15
Chinese vermicelli (soybean variety)	22	Onions (all kinds)	15
Eggplant	20	Peanuts	15
Fructose	20	Peppers (all colors and varieties)	15
Lemons	20	Spinach	15
Limes	20	Zucchini	15
Almonds; walnuts; hazelnuts	15	Avocados	10
Pecans	15		
Brazil nuts	15		

GI chart: alphabetical order

Dark chocolate (70 percent cocoa)	25	Lettuce (all kinds)	15
Eggplant	20	Maltose (beer)	110
Fennel	15	Melon*	60
Figs (dried)	40	Milk (1% low-fat or skim)	30
Figs (fresh)	35	Mung beans (soaked and cooked for 20 minutes)	30
Flour, white bread	85	Mushrooms	15
Fructose	20	Natural (unflavored) yogurt	35
Garlic	30	Nectarines	30
Glucose (dextrose)	100	Olives (all kinds)	15
Grapefruit	30	Onions (all kinds)	15
Grapes (all kinds)	45	Oranges	35
Herbs	15	Orange juice (commercial variety)	65
Honey	85	Orange juice (freshly squeezed)	45
Ice cream (made with alginates)	35	Pasta (made from whole wheat flour)	45
Jam (made with sugar)	65	Peaches	30
Jam (sugarfree)	30	Peanuts	15
Kidney beans	35	Pears	30
Kiwi	50	Peas, dried (cooked)	35
Leeks	15	Peas, fresh (cooked)	35
Lemons	20	Pecans	15
Limes	20	Peppers (all colors and varieties)	15
Lentils (brown)	30	Plums	35
Lentils (green)	25	Popcorn (no sugar added)	85
Lentils (red)	30	Potato chips	80
Lentils (yellow)	30	Potatoes (baked; skin on)	65

Potatoes (boiled; skin on)	65		Sorbet (sugarfree)	40
Potatoes (fried or french fried)	95		Sorbet (with sugar)	65
Potatoes (mashed)	80		Soybeans (cooked)	25
Potatoes (peeled; baked)	95		Spaghetti, durum wheat (cooked *al dente*)	40
Potatoes (peeled; boiled)	70		Spaghetti, whole wheat (cooked *al dente*)	40
Prunes	35		Spinach	15
Puffed rice	85		Split peas (yellow, cooked for 20 minutes)	25
Pumpkin*	75		Strawberries	25
Pumpkin seeds	15		Sugar (sucrose)	70
Pretzels	85		Sultanas	65
Raisins (dark or golden)	65		Sunflower seeds	15
Raspberries	25		Sweet potatoes	50
Ravioli; tortellini	70		Tapioca	85
Rice (brown)	50		Tomatoes	30
Rice (unrefined Basmati)	50		Turnips*	85
Rice cakes	85		Unrefined flour	50
Rice (long grain; white)	60		Unrefined flour, bread	40
Rice (pre-cooked)	90		Unrefined flour, pasta	40
Rice (pre-cooked; long grain)	70		Watermelon*	75
Risotto	70		White pasta, cooked well	55
Rye (whole wheat bread)	40		Whole wheat bread with bran	45
Quinoa	35		Wild rice	35
Satsumas	35		Zucchini	15
Semolina (white, cooked)	60			
Shortbread cookies	55			

Glossary

antioxidant
An enzyme or other organic molecule that can counteract the damaging effects of free radicals in the body.

AGI
Stands for the Average Glycemic Index, which is the resulting GI of two or more carbohydrates of differing GI values when eaten together.

carbohydrates
Also termed sugars, carbohydrates are the body's primary source of fuel. Carbohydrates are metabolized by the body into glucose, which acts as an important source of energy.

concentration of carbohydrates
The number of grams of carbohydrate a food contains per 100 gram (3.5-oz) serving.

diabetes type II
A chronic metabolic disorder that occurs when the body's cells become immune to insulin secreted by the pancreas. In many cases, the condition must be regulated with drugs.

discrepancy
A planned deviation from the diet that allows you to eat the occasional dessert, bag of chips, or any other food with a GI significantly higher than 50. You are allowed two discrepancies per month on the Weight Control Plan. Discrepancies are not allowed on the Rapid Weight Loss Plan.

fats
Complex molecules that store energy for long-term use by the body; also called fatty acids.

fructose
A naturally occurring fruit sugar with a low GI of 20. Fructose is thermostable, which means it retains its sweetness when heated and can be used in cooking and baking.

glucose
The sugar the body assimilates carbohydrates into; also a syrup made from cornstarch that is added to foods as a sweetener.

glycemia
The level of glucose in the blood; another term for blood sugar level.

glycemic index (GI)
A system that measures the amount of sugar a food contains and the effect it will have on blood sugar levels. Each food is assigned a number, which tells you comparatively, gram for gram, how much sugar a food contains, and how much of it will be absorbed by the body.

glycogen

Glucose that is converted into a short-term energy source and is stored in the muscles of the body. When blood sugar levels fall below normal, the body converts stored glycogen back into glucose.

hyperglycemia

An acute condition marked by extremely high blood sugar levels. This is caused by eating high-GI foods, which, in turn, triggers the pancreas to release a large amount of insulin to bring the blood sugar levels down to normal.

hyperinsulinism

A chronic metabolic condition in which the pancreas is very sensitive to glucose, releasing more—sometimes much more—insulin than is required in response to a carbohydrate.

hypoglycemia

An acute condition in which an excess of insulin in the blood causes abnormally low blood sugar levels. Symptoms include fatigue, lack of concentration, intense hunger, and irritability.

insulin

A hormone secreted by the pancreas, which chases sugar in the form of glucose out of the bloodstream and into the body's cells.

pancreas

An organ that produces enzymes that assist in digestion, along with hormones such as insulin, which helps the body use sugar for energy.

pastification

A mechanical process in which pasta dough is fed through small holes at a very high pressure. This gives the pastas, such as spaghetti, a protective film, which limits the amount of starch released during the cooking process and lowers the GI value by about five points.

protein

Organic substances that are found in a wide variety of animal and vegetable foods, particularly meat, fish, chicken, eggs, and soy products. Proteins contain large amounts of amino acids, which are used to make cells.

retrogradation

Also known as the cooling process, retrogradation can reduce the GI of some cooked carbohydrates, particularly pasta.

saturated fat

Saturated fat is solid at room temperature, and may contribute to cardiovascular disease. It is mainly derived from animal sources, such as fatty cuts of meat and butter.

unsaturated fat

Unsaturated fat is liquid at room temperature, and it does not contribute to cardiovascular disease. Some unsaturated fats (polyunsaturated fats, found mainly in fish) may even lower blood cholesterol levels. Unsaturated fats are derived mainly from vegetable sources, such as olive oil, and oily fish, such as salmon and tuna.

Useful resources

General information

www.montignac.com

The Montignac Universal Official Website, complete with detailed information about the science behind the diet, extensive GI listings, Montignac product information, and a forum for questions and advice about the diet.

For natural and organic foods

Whole Foods Market is the world's largest retailer of natural and organic foods, including Arabica coffee, whole grain bread, whole wheat pasta, seeds, nuts, sugar-free fruit preserves, and a wide variety of beans, grains, and fructose. There are over 155 Whole Foods Markets throughout North America and the United Kingdom, www.wholefoodsmarket.com

For low-carbohydrate, low GI food products

www.locarbu.com/

For specialty foods

Gourmet Garage
www.gourmetgarage.com

Dean & Deluca
www.deandeluca.com

Eli's Vinegar Factory
www.elismanhattan.com
(212) 987-0885

Fresh Direct
www.freshdirect.com

www.HealthyGourmetStore.com

For buying goose fat

www.ChefShop.com

For foie gras, paté, duck confit, etc.

Frenchy Bee Gourmet
www.frenchybee.com

For game meat, foie gras, paté, and speciality sausages, etc.

D'Artagnan
www.dartagnan.com

Information on diabetes

American Diabetes Association
1701 North Beauregard Street
Alexandria, VA 22311
Tel: (800) DIABETES
www.diabetes.org

National Institute of Diabetes
and Digestive and Kidney Diseases
1 Information Way
Bethesda, MD 20892-3560
Tel: 1-800-860-8747
www.diabetes.niddk.nih.gov

Information on a healthy diet

American Dietetic Association

1201 South Riverside Plaza

Suite 2000

Chicago, IL 60606-6995

Tel: (800) 877-1600

www.eatright.org

National Agricultural Library

Food and Nutrition Information Center

10301 Baltimore Avenue

Beltsville, MD 20705-2351

www.nutrition.gov

Information on organic food

Organic Consumers Association

6101 Cliff Estate Road

Little Marais, MN 55614

Tel: (218) 226-4164

www.organicconsumers.org

Recommended reading by the same author

Eat Yourself Slim

(Alex & Lucas Publishing, 2004)

The Montignac Method Just for Children

(Montignac Publishing Ltd, 2004)

Montignac Provençal Cookbook

(Montignac Publishing Ltd, 2002)

The Miracle of Wine

(Montignac Publishing Ltd, 1997)

Dine Out and Lose Weight

(Montignac Publishing Ltd, 1996)

The Montignac Method Just for Women

(Montignac Publishing Ltd, 1995)

Montignac Recipes and Menus

(Montignac Publishing Ltd, 1993)

Index

Acknowledgments

AUTHOR'S ACKNOWLEDGMENTS

Michel Montignac would like to say a special thanks to: Suzy, my darling wife who graciously gave up parties and weekends during the writing of this book to help me find the appropriate words and expressions; Mónica Lalinde, my assistant, whose computer expertise was especially valuable to me as I am still a beginner in this area; Ernest Hilton, the manager and owner of the Montignac Boutique & Café (gourmet food store, café, and wine bar at 160 Old Brompton Road, London, UK), who has become an expert on my diet, and who supplied the recipes for this book; Shannon Beatty, my editor at DK, who spent many late nights and weekends working on this project; Jenny Jones at DK, who also devoted a great deal of her time to this book; Jo Grey for the beautiful book design; and Mary-Clare Jerram for her unwavering support for this book.

PUBLISHER'S ACKNOWLEDGMENTS

Dorling Kindersley would like to thank Kate Whitaker for photography; Luis Peral for art direction; home economist Valerie Berry for making the recipes camera-ready; Penny Markham for the styling; Siobhan O'Connor for editing the recipes; Ernest Hilton for providing the recipes; Diana Vowles for additional editorial assistance; Christine Heilman for editing the Canadian edition; Valerie Chandler for compiling the index, and Wes Martin and Barbara Bowman for their enormous help in making the recipes U.S.-ready.

Picture credits

Laurie Evans 10–11, 25, 30–31, 33, 47, 58–59, 68–69, 238–39
Corbis: 27, 76–77, 98–99, 134–35
All other images © DK Images

About the Author

Michel Montignac, world-renowned diet expert, was born in southern France. Dealing with the daily challenge of fattening business lunches while working for a large pharmaceutical firm led him to study nutrition. After years of studying metabolism, he developed the "Montignac Method," a unique diet plan based on the glycemic index that enabled him to lose 35 pounds in three months. Montignac's book *Eat Yourself Slim* became a multimillion-copy international bestseller. He is the author of over 20 books, which are available in more than 42 countries and 25 languages. Montignac lives in Geneva and devotes his time to research, writing, and lecturing.

For more information, visit www.montignac.com